# *MAP: The Co-Creative White Brotherhood Medical Assistance Program*

THIRD EDITION

# MAP

# THE CO-CREATIVE WHITE BROTHERHOOD MEDICAL ASSISTANCE PROGRAM

MACHAELLE SMALL WRIGHT

*PERELANDRA, LTD.*

*CENTER FOR NATURE RESEARCH*

*JEFFERSONTON · VIRGINIA*

Second Edition 1994
THIRD EDITION 2006


For information, write Perelandra, Ltd.


This book is manufactured in the United States of America.
Designed by Machaelle Wright.
Cover design by James F. Brisson, Williamsville, VT 05362.
Editing by David and Machaelle Wright.
Copyediting by Elizabeth McHale, Williamsburg, MA 01096.
Proofreading and GROMS extraordinaire:
Beth Shelton, Jeannette Edwards and Joyce McVey.
Food: Maria Gabriel.
Formatting, typesetting, and computer wizardry
by Machaelle Small Wright.
This book was formatted, laid out and
produced using QuarkXPress software.
Printed on recycled paper.
Published by Perelandra, Ltd., Warrenton, VA 20188

Library of Congress Control Number: 2006933118
Wright, Machaelle Small
*MAP: The Co-Creative White Brotherhood Medical Assistance Program*
ISBN 0-927978-62-8

6 8 9 7

# *Contents*

*Preface*

# *The Light at the End of the Tunnel*

## *by Albert Schatz, Ph.D.*

THIS IS AN EXTRAORDINARY BOOK. To do it justice, I would like to begin by putting it in proper perspective. Man's localized destruction of nature has been responsible for the extinction of many animal species. Now our global assault on nature threatens *our* survival. Instead of implementing Franklin Delano Roosevelt's Four Freedoms, we have chosen a collision course with the Four Horsemen of the Apocalypse. Individuals who exhibit such self-destructive behavior are considered to be mentally deranged. But, like Thespians in a Greek tragedy, "merrily we go to hell."

We are running out of natural resources, out of natural environment, out of space, and out of time. In our suicidal assault on nature, we are approaching the point of no return. The world's military budget is a barometer, odometer, and speedometer of our mad rush to oblivion. The arms race turns out to have been a race to annihilation. The insanity of Vietnam has metastasized into global insanity. In Vietnam, "we had to destroy a city in order to save it." Now we are destroying the world

—allegedly to save it in one way or another, for one purpose or another. The wages of this sin were pointed out by Dwight Eisenhower in his 1953 Cross of Iron speech.

> *... Every gun that is made, every warship launched, every rocket fired signifies, in the final sense, a theft from those who hunger and are not fed, those who are cold and are not clothed.*
>
> *This world in arms is not spending money alone.*
>
> *It is spending the sweat of its laborers, the genius of its scientists, the hopes of its children.*
>
> *The cost of one modern heavy bomber is this: a modern brick school in more than thirty cities....*
>
> *We pay for a single fighter plane with a half million bushels of wheat.*
>
> *We pay for a single destroyer with new homes that could have housed more than eight thousand people.*
>
> *This, I repeat, is the best way of life to be found on the road the world has been taking.*
>
> *This is not a way of life at all, in any true sense. Under the cloud of threatening war, it is humanity hanging from a cross of iron....*

We obviously will not be saved by our anthropocentric science, which has given us chemical dumps, deadly radioactive waste that we do not know how to dispose of, air and water pollution, carcinogenic pesticides and food additives, ineffective and harmful synthetic drugs, nerve gas, nuclear weapons, biological warfare, the profligate waste of natural resources, the global devastation of nature, and much more. This is what science means to many people. We obviously also will not be saved by academic scientists whose research is supported by grants from and, in turn, supports the pharmaceutical, agricultural, and chemical industries—and the military. The military-industrial complex that Eisenhower warned us about has metastasized into a military-industrial-educational complex.

## YE SHALL KNOW THE TRUTH AND THE TRUTH SHALL MAKE YOU FREE

Where can we go from here? Is there a way out? I am convinced that our only salvation is what Machaelle Small Wright calls "co-creative science." This involves our consciously establishing a co-creative partnership with nature. But before we do that, we should know what nature is and who we are with respect to nature.

This and other essential information is now readily available as a result of research that Machaelle has done in collaboration with nature. Her published reports are not merely descriptive narratives of devas, nature spirits, and other intelligences. Instead, they provide us with clear definitions and a simple hands-on approach so we know how and with whom we can communicate and work. Moreover, we can all engage in co-creative science and work in a co-creative partnership with nature, *if* we want to. It is not necessary that we take courses in biology, chemistry, physics, geology, calculus, etc., and get degrees. The only credentials we need are intent, sincerity, commitment, and the information and processes available to us in Perelandra publications.

Co-creative science is qualitatively different from the science we know because it integrates the involutionary dynamic of nature (order, organization, and life vitality/action) with the evolutionary dynamic of man (definition, direction and purpose). Until now, science has been essentially evolutionary. Co-creative science is therefore not a linear advance over present-day science, but it is qualitatively unique. It was developed *de novo* in the sense that it is not derived from contemporary science. It employs different methodologies and obtains information from sources with which contemporary science has never worked. Co-creative science may be graphically represented, using the "V" diagram shown on the next page.

I believe that co-creative science is the science of the future, that it will revolutionize our understanding of science, philosophy, and psychology; and that it will provide us with a new kind of agriculture and new ways of achieving health.

This leads directly to Machaelle Wright's book—*MAP: The Co-Creative White Brotherhood Medical Assistance Program.* All of us are concerned with health. But what is health? And how is it best achieved, supported, and maintained? Unfortunately, there is something wrong with how these questions are answered. While we have been bombarded with more and more information on health, our health has been declining. While we have been spending more and more money on health, we have become more and more unhealthy. Obviously, what we need is a new approach, one that will be effective. *MAP* provides precisely that.

MAP is not allopathy, homeopathy, naturopathy, or any other conventional medical specialty. Nor is it related to alternative health modalities or holistic health. And it is not esoteric, occult, new age, or spiritual. All those approaches to health are essentially evolutionary developments by man.

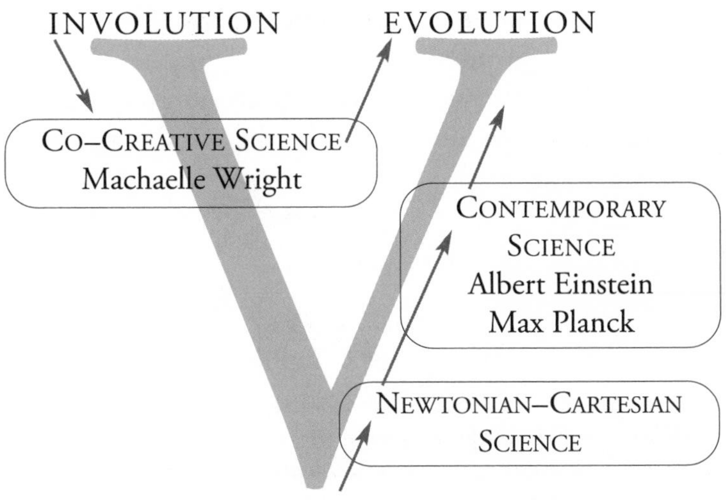


*Newtonian–Cartesian Science, also known as Classical Science, developed in the 17th century. That science was based on the work of the physicist Sir Isaac Newton and the philosopher René Descartes. Contemporary, present-day science is based on the research of Max Planck, "the father of quantum mechanics" (1900), and Albert Einstein's theories of relativity (1905 and 1916).*

---

MAP is qualitatively different because, like co-creative science of which it is a part, it integrates the involutionary input of nature with man's evolutionary development. The healthy human being is a balanced combination of these two dynamics. We do not need to know anatomy, physiology, biochemistry, pathology, psychology, etc., to use MAP effectively. As in the case of co-creative science, the only credentials we need are intent, sincerity, commitment, and the information and processes in Machaelle's book.

But *MAP* offers much more than just health *per se.* Like Machaelle's other books, *MAP* also increases our understanding of who and what we are, what nature and reality are, what our place in the universe is, what our responsibilities are, and what amazing opportunities we have.

Machaelle's co-creative research with nature is not only the light at the end of the tunnel. It is also the entrance to the tunnel and the tunnel itself.

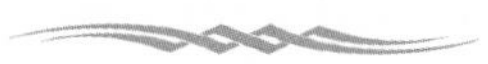

*Dr. Schatz discovered the antibiotic Streptomycin, which was the first effective means of treating human tuberculosis. For this and other research, he received honorary degrees and medals, and was named an honorary member of medical, dental and scientific societies in Europe, Latin America and the U.S.*

# *MAP: The Co-Creative White Brotherhood Medical Assistance Program*

# *L'Chaim*

*Chapter 1*

# *Some Personal Comments and How MAP Was Developed*

IN 1982, MY WORK EXPANDED in ways that were both exhilarating and extremely challenging. Since 1976, I had been working exclusively with nature intelligence in research dedicated to developing a working partnership between humans and nature. But in 1982, I learned from nature that I could expand the research in a way that would link it directly into the activities of an organization called the "White Brotherhood." I also learned that this connection was beneficial to nature and to us, as well as to the White Brotherhood. So, I decided to do it.

This decision set off a chain of events that, among other things, led me into a whole new level of understanding of the human body and its relationship to the soul. You see, my decision to expand the research at Perelandra was a soul decision. Once the decision was made, I discovered that implementing it depended on my ability to physically hold, support and process all that the expansion required of me. I had understood something about this relationship between the soul and the body for years, but the 1982 expansion brought it into a new and more intense light.

Usually, when I've discussed this situation with others, they immediately think that the thing one must do in order to meet the challenges of expansion is change the diet. Over the years, I've realized how much we lean on diet as a solution for everything. Well, I never changed my diet nor, after much questioning, was I instructed to change my diet. The eating patterns that I had established prior to 1982 were sufficient for what I was faced with after 1982. If diet wasn't the answer to my functioning well on this expanded level of the nature research, then I would have to find other answers.

To help you to understand the scope of the expansion I am talking about and why it presented challenges, let me give you a thumbnail description of the White Brotherhood and nature intelligence. After all, if you decide to enter the MAP program, you will be working with them as well and I'm sure you'd appreciate knowing who they are. But before you get nervous and think that your working with them will necessitate your dealing with the kinds of challenges I encountered, let me assure you that this will not be the case. I had to expand myself into the dimension of the White Brotherhood in order to work with them on a daily basis in a working team relationship. This has impacted the scope, quality, direction and expression of the Perelandra work.* Your expansion will center around your decision to work with the White Brotherhood and nature in areas involving your health and personal balance. You will not have to expand into another dimension. In short, the White Brotherhood and nature team will be making "house calls."

---

* *I wrote about this expansion and the work that resulted from it in two books,* Dancing in the Shadows of the Moon *and* The Mount Shasta Mission.

## THE WHITE BROTHERHOOD

I became aware of the White Brotherhood's link with the research at Perelandra in 1980. For two years, I ignored them while I maintained my focus exclusively on nature intelligence and our work. I figured that whatever connection the White Brotherhood had would be best handled by them and they did not need me. Besides, at that time, I knew next to nothing about them and had no desire to know more.

Much has been written about the White Brotherhood, but I think a lot of it was garbage. Some people have felt or said that they were the sole "channellers" of the White Brotherhood, and this simply isn't true. The Brotherhood is a huge organization that is constantly connected to us in general and to many of us individually. It's just that usually they are only able to work with us on an intuitive level, and our link with them is unconscious on our part.

The White Brotherhood is a large group of highly evolved souls dedicated to assisting the evolutionary process of moving universal reality, principles, laws and patterns through all planes and levels of form. They hold the major patterning and rhythms now being utilized for the shift we are all going through from the Piscean to the Aquarian era. When we link with them, they support and assist us by assuring that any work we do maintains its forward evolutionary motion and its connection to the new Aquarian dynamics.

They exist beyond time and history. I first heard about them during my stay at the Findhorn community in Scotland in 1977. St. Germain, who had a close relationship with several Findhorn members, was referred to often and described as being a master teacher from the White Brotherhood. I was also told that the Order of the Melchizedek was a part of the Brotherhood, and it is from this group that all of the major religious leaders come who have been a part of our history. As I have said, I ignored the Brotherhood and its existence for years, assuming that they knew how to do their job, whatever that was, very well without me and that my focus was primarily on nature, not on human-oriented evolution. After all, this is the age of specialization.

My understanding of how the Brotherhood functions is, I'm sure, somewhat simplistic. I see them operating in a cooperative role with us on this planet. They design and infuse purpose and direction into the frameworks of social order through which we on Earth move in order to learn, experience and evolve. In essence, they create the schools through which we move. We call these schools religions, governmental structures, educational movements, philosophy, science . . . all those massive social frameworks with which we associate and within which we function.

Let me say something about the name "White Brotherhood." Since publishing *MAP* in 1990, several people have written me questioning—and sometimes complaining about—that name. They want to make sure this isn't some white supremacist or sexist organization before buying *MAP* and getting into the program. Trust me, the White Brotherhood is neither. It includes males, females and souls beyond both persuasions, and they can outdo us any day when it comes to color.

The name "White Brotherhood" has been used for this group for centuries. We did not coin the name here at Perelandra. It was coined by those folks on the Earth level who first began to consciously work with this group. It is not a name the Brotherhood chose for itself. It is a name we chose for it. The words "white brotherhood" maintained the integrity and intent of the group, so it has always been acceptable to them. "White" is used to signify *all* the rays of the light spectrum. "Brotherhood" is used to signify not only the family of all *people* but also the family of all *life*.

If the name sticks in your throat and causes you a problem in deciding whether or not you would like to participate in MAP, here's what I suggest. Put aside your objections temporarily. Start the program and allow yourself enough time to get comfortably settled in. This should take four to six weeks, at most. Once you are settled, address your objections to the name "White Brotherhood." If you still have objections, consider what name you would feel comfortable with that would maintain the intent of this vast group. Ask your MAP team if your name is acceptable to use when you are referring to this group. Unless you are way off base with your name, I'm sure they will have no objections. They will just need to know that when *you* say "Purple Peoplehood" or "Neutral Androgynyhood," you mean them.

One other point: Your special name for the White Brotherhood is between you and them. It would be neither helpful nor accurate to feel your name is for everyone and announce it to others. Not all of us have a problem with the name nor do we seek to change it. It would be more helpful to allow others to make their own decisions and work on their own with their team around this issue.

## NATURE

As I mentioned earlier, my work with the White Brotherhood focuses on nature. The Medical Assistance Program (MAP) is an example of the Brotherhood and nature working together for our benefit within an organized framework that we call MAP: The Co-Creative White Brotherhood Medical Assistance Program.

The keystone of MAP is its coning. It is set up to assure perfect balance between the involution dynamic (nature) and the evolution dynamic (the White Brotherhood and you). The evolution dynamic supplies the definition, direction and purpose to any thing or action. The involution dynamic (nature) supplies the matter, means and action for achieving evolution's definition, direction and purpose. The human soul is the force behind the evolution dynamic. Nature is the force behind involution. In health, the evolution dynamic comes from one's soul. And it is from our soul that we receive the impulses that define our direction and purpose. It is the soul that gives the necessary data to nature for all that is physically required for a human to fully operate within a given lifetime. Nature then supplies us our body according to these soul-directed specifications. This also means that nature is the engineer of the human body and, like any good engineer, knows how it is supposed to work and how to fix it if it isn't working correctly.

In MAP, nature also anchors the program and makes it accessible to everyone on our level as well as to the medical teams in the White Brotherhood. Because of nature, we need not have an intermediary third party bridging us into the White Brotherhood. Nature's presence allows the medical teams to work with us directly.

Now, there are some fine books written about nature intelligence, how to communicate with them and how to work with them. I know this because I wrote some of them! I may not have been familiar with the White Brotherhood when MAP was begun, but I was sure familiar with nature. I don't want to bog you down with a boatload of information about nature or conings. But, to help with your understanding, I have included several definitions in this section and a section in the Appendices (Appendix A) on conings. If you wish to understand more about nature intelligence in general, I recommend the book *Co-Creative Science: A Revolution in Science Providing Real Solutions for Today's Health and Environment*

The following is a good working definition of nature. In fact, it is what nature gave me when I asked it to define key terms it uses often in the Perelandra research and work. (The full definitions by nature are reprinted in Appendix E.)

● NATURE. *In the larger universe and beyond, on its many levels and dimensions, there are a number of groups of consciousnesses that, although equal in importance, are quite different in expression and function.... Together, they make up the full expression of the larger, total life picture. No one piece, no one expression, can be missing or the larger life picture on all its levels and dimensions will cease to exist. One such consciousness has been universally termed "nature." Because of what we are saying about the larger picture not existing without all of its parts, you may assume that nature as both a reality and a consciousness exists on all dimensions and all levels. It cannot be excluded.*

*Each group of consciousnesses has what can be termed an area of expertise. As we said, all groups are equal in importance but express and function differently from one another. These different expressions and functions are vital to the overall balance of reality. A truly symbiotic relationship exists among the groups and is based on balance—universal balance. . . . Nature is a massive, intelligent consciousness group that expresses and functions within the many areas of involution—that is, moving soul-oriented consciousness into any dimension or level of form.*

*Nature is the conscious reality that supplies order, organization and life vitality for this shift. Nature is the consciousness that is, for your working understanding, intimately linked with form. Nature is the consciousness that comprises all form on all levels and dimensions. It* is *form's order, organization and life vitality. Nature is first and foremost a consciousness of equal importance with all other consciousnesses in the largest scheme of reality. It expresses and functions uniquely in that it comprises all form on all levels and dimensions and is responsible for and creates all of form's order, organization and life vitality.*

To assist you in understanding "nature," I include nature's definitions of form, deva and nature spirit.

● FORM. *We consider reality to be in the form state when there is order, organization and life vitality combined with a state of consciousness. . . .*

*We do not consider form to be only that which is perceptible to the five senses. In fact, we see form from this perspective to be most limited, both in its life reality and in its ability to function. We see form from the perspective of the five senses to be useful only for the most basic and fundamental level of identification. From this perspective, there is very little relationship to the full understanding and knowledge of how a unit or form system functions.*

*All energy contains order, organization and life vitality; therefore, all energy is form. . . .*

*On planet Earth, the character, personality, emotional makeup, intellectual capacity, strong points and gifts of a human are all form. They are that which gives order, organization and life vitality to consciousness.*

*Order and organization are the physical structures that create a framework for form. They define the walls. But we have included the dynamic of life vitality when we refer to form because one of the elements of form is action, and it is life vitality that initiates and creates action.*

● DEVA AND NATURE SPIRIT. *"Deva" and "nature spirit" are names used to identify two different levels and functions within the nature consciousness. They are the two levels within the larger nature consciousness that interface with the human soul while in form. There are other levels, and they are differentiated from one another primarily by specific expression and function.*

*To expand from our definition of form, it is the devic level that fuses with consciousness to create order, organization and life vitality. The devic level as the architect designs the complex order, organization and life vitality that will be needed by the soul consciousness while functioning within the scope or band of form. If the consciousness chooses to shift from one point of form to another point, thereby changing form function, it is the devic level of nature that alters the order, organization and life vitality accordingly. The devic level designs and is the creation of the order, organization and life vitality of form.*

*The nature spirit level infuses the devic order, organization and life vitality and adds to this the dynamic of function and working balance. To order, organization and life vitality it brings move-*

*ment and the bond that maintains the alignment of the devic form unit to the universal principles of balance while the consciousness is in form.*

*To say that nature is the expert in areas of form and form principles barely scratches the surface of the true nature (pardon the pun) of nature's role in form. It is the expert of form, and it is form itself. A soul-oriented consciousness cannot exist on any level or dimension of form in any way without an equal, intimate, symbiotic relationship with the nature consciousness.*

For you to work with MAP, you will be working with the White Brotherhood plus two different levels of nature intelligence: the devic and the nature spirit levels. As stated in the above definition, these two names, "deva" and "nature spirit," are used to identify two different expressions and functions within the nature consciousness. The specific areas of nature intelligence you will be working with in MAP are the Deva of Healing and Pan.

● Deva of healing. As part of the devic level, this intelligence functions as an architectural force and creates the physical structures found within all human healing. The order, organization and life vitality of the human body—that is, the full physical structure and how it functions—fall within the domain of the Deva of Healing. Since MAP is focused on the health and balance of us humans, it is critical that the nature intelligence responsible for the physical process of healing the human body be included in the coning. With its presence, the White Brotherhood is assured that all healing processes within MAP maintain the integrity of natural law to its fullest.

● PAN. "Pan" is the traditional name for the nature spirit level that oversees and coordinates the full nature spirit level. I call Pan the CEO of the nature spirit level. The devic level *creates* all of the blueprints for form. The nature spirit level *implements* those blueprints—it is the builder. It also coordinates the action and movement of all form and ensures that this activity maintains the integrity of the original devic blueprint. In MAP, Pan aligns all physical elements of any action or process that might occur in a session to the devic healing blueprint.

We work with Pan in MAP because it/he is the only nature spirit element that does not have regional limitations. He is universal in dynamic. This means that everyone, no matter where they are positioned on the planet, can work with Pan. His universality is critical for a program that was intended to be global. (By the way, Pan is actually without, or beyond, gender. I refer to him as "him" because his energy feels masculine to me during our communications.)

Finally, it is the nature spirit level, represented by Pan, that keys our physical presence into the medical units of the White Brotherhood and stabilizes that presence during the session.

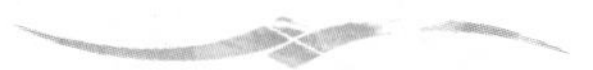

Let me tell you a little about how this program came into existence. As I have mentioned, the expansion of my work with nature into this new level of teamwork with the Brotherhood required that I physically shift and operate in new ways that would support and process the new level of work. It was such a massive jump for me that my body systems did not know how to adjust to the new demands. The first thing that occurred was that I began to misalign structurally. I had worked with a chiropractor for years previous to this as part of my general maintenance health program, and I knew my body was structurally strong. I rarely needed a chiropractic adjustment. Now I needed them once or twice a month, and the adjustments were fairly extensive. At first, I said nothing to my chiropractor about the new level of work. But, after the first visit, she mentioned that something was odd. I was suddenly requiring a lot of adjustments and not requiring flower essences. (She routinely includes flower essence testing in her work.) Normally, when she sees the scope of adjustments I was needing, they are emotionally induced and require flower essences stabilization. I was not testing positive for the essences. Though she didn't voice them, she was beginning to have questions.

After the second visit, during which I required as many adjustments as the first, I told her briefly what I was doing and something about its effect on my work and life. She didn't even blink. She just said that explained what she was seeing. My body didn't know how to process what I was now working with and it was "flying out of alignment" from the strain. I would need periodic adjustments while my body system was learning how to function within the new level of reality.

The second major problem I had to face was the sudden development of head pain. I felt as if my head wanted to explode. It wasn't a conventional headache—it was more like somebody had an air hose hooked up to my head and was pumping in air well beyond the capacity that my head could hold.

I returned to the chiropractor and told her about the head pressure. Luckily, she was one of five percent of chiropractors in the United States who were trained in cranial adjustments.

My physical system had to pick up these new impulses and translate them accurately in order to process what was happening to me, perceive accurately what I was working with, and function well within that perception. All this is accomplished primarily within the sacrum, spinal column and cranials, and it directly impacts the flow and pulsations of the cerebrospinal fluid. It is also along the spinal column that impulses are first processed by the nervous system. We could see by the adjustments I needed that all of this new action was having an impact on my sacrum, spine and head. The body, not knowing how to receive such a massive infusion of impulses or how to translate this input accurately, reacted by either overloading or closing down. Physically, this would result in misalignment of the sacrum, vertebrae, and/or misalignment or jamming of the cranials. The skull is composed of ten major cranial bones that expand and contract according to the ebb and flow of the cerebrospinal fluid. The massive infusion of new impulses was akin to throwing a monkey wrench into this normal physical operation and knocking things out of kilter. Hence, the head pain.

My chiropractor and I worked together to assist my body in shifting to a different structural alignment that would better facilitate the new work I was doing. I could then learn how to process the new impulses with ease and accuracy. For a year and a half, we worked together. We responded to the glitches as they occurred (these were easy for me to detect since they resulted in various degrees of pain). The chiropractor was smart enough not to dictate what alignment I should be in; rather, she observed what alignment my body was moving toward and assisted that movement.

Our work was brought to a climax after a year and a half

when my parietal cranials moved into what the chiropractor called a "parietal spread." These two massive bones at the top of the skull assumed a position allowing their expansion and contraction to operate within a new, expanded range. With this, the head pain was relieved. The chiropractor said she felt that all of our work over the past year and a half had led to this one major adjustment. We both felt that our work together had gone as far as it could go.

For a few months, all was well. But in the summer of 1984, the head pain returned. I remember I was in the garden when I realized that my head was beginning to hurt. I guess, as is often the case in these moments of change, I felt my work with the chiropractor was no longer feasible for practical reasons. Her office is an hour and a half drive, and her practice is so large that I often had to wait a week or two for an appointment. For some reason, none of this had made any difference to me when I went to her previously. But now it was unacceptable. I felt I could not wait to have this head pain alleviated, and I was unwilling to continue driving such a long distance for what I now thought would be never-ending treatment.

A thought popped into my mind. Perhaps the White Brotherhood could somehow be of assistance. With my head pain increasing, I figured it was worth a shot. I connected with the White Brotherhood, told them my problem, and asked if there was something they could do to help me. They told me to lie down, open a coning (to be explained later), and they would connect me with help. I followed their instructions—and met Lorpuris, the head of the White Brotherhood Medical Unit.

I explained to Lorpuris what my physical discomforts were and tried to describe them as fully as I could. He instructed me to just lie quietly and comfortably, and he then set to work. The session lasted about an hour, during which I felt as if I was getting an energy charge or current through different parts of my body. It wasn't painful at all, but I must admit that it was so different from anything I had ever felt that I found the sensations to be both exciting and a little scary. At the end of the hour, Lorpuris suggested that we meet regularly so that I could go through comprehensive body balancing to facilitate my new level of operation. I agreed and we "made a date." When I closed down the session and walked back outside, I realized that my head no longer hurt. I was amazed.

Since 1984, Lorpuris and I have continued to meet regularly. In the process of helping me physically and emotionally to adjust to my ever-expanding work and life, we explored various ways in which he and his extensive medical unit could work with others here on Earth in areas of health and healing. In fact, they had been interested in making this kind of connection with us for some time.

But there were two major problems that had to be surmounted in order for us to successfully work with the White Brotherhood Medical Unit. First, there was the problem of their keying into our life system on all levels (physical, emotional, mental and spiritual) and maintaining that connection with us clearly and long enough for a medical session. We solved this problem by bringing nature on board as a member of the Brotherhood team. When I connect with my medical team, I do it within a coning, a vortex of energy that includes nature intelligence, the medical team and me. Within this coning vortex, nature is able to stabilize us on all levels with the Brotherhood.

The second problem involved communication between us and our medical team. They did not want to establish a working relationship that would exclude all but the few who knew how to receive interlevel communication. We solved this problem in two ways. The MAP sessions have built into them schedules and time frames that enable everyone to utilize the program even if they are unable to sense or hear anything from their team. All people have to do is follow the MAP instructions and the schedule. They don't have to hear from their team when they should meet with them or for how long. This is already spelled out for them. All they have to do is talk—tell the team what is going on with them and what is out of sorts. The team can hear us effortlessly even if we can't hear them. The other solution to the communication problem was kinesiology. Those who want to ask questions and receive answers from their team can do so by using a simple yes/no format. Then, they can "read" the answers from their team by kinesiology testing. This opens the communication door from both sides. (See Appendix B for how to do kinesiology.)

Another point about communication: When we first enter MAP, we may not be able to hear or sense our team. (But we will sense things happening to us physically from time to time during the sessions.) As we continue the program, we will become used to our team, be better able to process the input from them, and we will have gone through some of the clearing and adjustments necessary for us to sense our team, and not just experience their work. As for actually hearing our team? Over the many years since *MAP* was first published, most people tell me that they never hear their team and that it doesn't matter. They can still get their questions answered using kinesiology and they definitely feel the differences in the quality of their health.

We have cleared up the two major stumbling blocks, and as a result MAP was created. The shingle has been hung. The office is now open. And you are invited to enter the program.

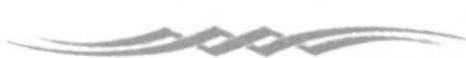

*Chapter 2*

# *How MAP Can Help You*

TO GIVE YOU AN IDEA OF HOW MAP came into my life, I have talked about a somewhat exceptional development that most people would not encounter in their lives, but that was responsible for leading me into MAP. However, I don't want to leave the impression that MAP is only for exceptional times. It is not. MAP is for those who feel that their present medical support—whether traditional or alternative—is not enough. For years, you may have felt absolutely comfortable with your medical support, and then suddenly, without a shadow of a doubt, you know you need more. To function *well* you need more input, more support. Yet, when you look around and try alternatives, none feel right. MAP is then your answer.

Because the MAP team includes nature, MAP is a *physical* program (not a spiritual program) that works on your well-being from the physical, emotional, mental and spiritual perspectives. Because of the unique position of the MAP team, it works on strains, pressures, pain and conflict being felt on all these levels *simultaneously.* When it comes to our health issues, these four levels interrelate. Normally we go to professionals who are experts in one level or one area of a level. It is up to us to put a team together that addresses the different aspects of the problem. And, when we put these teams together, they rarely consult with one another. So we don't have a sense of a united and coordinated medical approach. The MAP teams work on all levels simultaneously and function as a coordinated unit. Consequently, a MAP session is more comprehensive and its results are deeper than those of other health systems.

We can initiate MAP during times of illness and injury, or it can be initiated during times of relative health when we feel we are capable of a better level of health and balance—and we want it. MAP is a comprehensive health program that you will use throughout your entire life. It is not a one-time program only for emergency situations. We are constantly changing and developing throughout our lives. MAP helps us maintain a high level of balance and function throughout all our changes and shifts. In short, it gives us a chance to experience an exceptional quality of life.

We can begin MAP at any stage in our life and at any age. We do not have to be healthy to begin (some have thought this was necessary), and we do not have to be sick. We do not need to abandon any medical support we have been using in order to begin MAP. If you are combining other health practices with MAP, this is fine. Just tell your MAP team what other things you include and how. MAP will accommodate them. As I worked with my team and experienced the depth of their work, I gradually dropped the other health practices I had been using, one by one. Before I felt comfortable switching my medical needs to MAP exclusively, my confidence about MAP had to grow. However, if I had a serious illness or injury that needed quick medical attention, I would not hesitate to get it. The difference is that I would work with my MAP team throughout the "repair" and recuperation period, as well.

It is important that you understand one thing about working with a White Brotherhood MAP team. *They will not, under any circumstances, circumvent your timing on any issue.* You are in complete control and command of your timing and rate of development. They will not circumvent your timing, because it would be wrong to do so. This would, in effect, remove you from the driver's seat in your own life and place you in the position of a child being catered to by the almighty parent. Your team will simply not participate in such activity.

In MAP, *you* control your timing and development in an interesting way. You will note in the instructions that you are urged to talk to your team. Tell them everything that comes to mind that is bothering you on any of your PEMS levels (physical, emotional, mental and spiritual). You aren't going through this exercise because your team is stupid and can't see you are in trouble. The troubles or situations you can articulate to your team tell them what you are ready to work on. And the extent to which you can describe the situation tells them the extent to which you are ready to change what is bothering you. *You are your own barometer.* They will not work in areas beyond those you recognize and describe. Consequently, your team will never put you in a position of facing and dealing with something for which you are unprepared. In the MAP sessions, *you* are your own master, and your team assists you in achieving your goals of health and balance in ways that are beyond belief. You are simply demonstrating your wisdom by choosing the best team with which to work.

## SESSION: LORPURIS

*I would like to add a bit to what Machaelle has already written. In short, I would like to assure you that we are eager to assist you in your quest for health and balance in any way you see fit. There will be those who will gravitate to MAP and wish to establish themselves in the program, but they will hesitate because they will feel unworthy of such an expanded approach or feel inferior, believing that we would consider it bothersome to work with them. It is this situation I would like to address.*

*I would like to point out that it is not a sign of good health and balance if individuals refuse help despite the fact they have gravitated toward the very help they are refusing. You might feel that I am stating the obvious. But we see the greatest stumbling block in establishing the kind of medical assistance that so many are presently seeking, either consciously or unconsciously, as being this issue of feeling unworthy of the help. It is a vicious cycle—and one we cannot step in from "out of the blue" and release a person from.*

*We suggest that if the concept of MAP feels right to you, yet you are feeling hesitant because you can't believe something "so good" could come to you, that you temporarily put aside your hesitancies for the purpose of entering the program. As we have said, feeling unworthy—and I use the word "unworthy" to cover feelings such as inferiority, weakness, fear and lack of capability—is a sign of being in need of help. Once you have entered the program and have discussed with us the reasons for your hesitancies, we will then be able to work with you to obtain a new level of balance that will effectively adjust your sense of self-worth and thus take care of the very reason you might not have entered the program.*

In the MAP workshops I have given at Perelandra, this issue of self-worth has come up often. Invariably, someone will say he or she simply can't understand why a medical team from the White Brotherhood would choose to work with them. And, if the White Brotherhood does this kind of work with them, doesn't it mean that they are being chosen by the Brotherhood to then do something significant—like save the world or something? Surely you can't remain "just a housewife" or a car mechanic if you have a MAP team.

In the overall picture, the White Brotherhood is presently focused on shifting all that exists on this planet from a Piscean dynamic (parent/child) to an Aquarian dynamic (teamwork). Everything must shift. And all of us are involved in this shift. No one is exempt. We are responsible for catching on to what's happening and doing the work needed to make this shift. The MAP medical teams are not doing something extraordinary for a handful of "chosen" people. This program is for everyone who wants it. By working with us individually, the MAP teams assist us in living life with a better balance and getting on with the changes that are needed. Everything that is involved in the work of a housewife or auto mechanic must go through this shift, as well. The last thing a MAP team wants you to do is throw away everything and go off to "save the world." MAP wants you to do what you are meant to do, do it the best you can, and take responsibility for shifting your piece of the life puzzle from the Piscean picture to the Aquarian picture. It's all important to MAP. No one is insignificant.

## EXPANDED EXPERIENCES AND MAP

Since the MAP program developed as a response to my struggles with integrating an expanded level of operation, I asked Lorpuris to explain how we operate during times of expansion.

Now, don't get confused here. MAP is for general health balance, regular health issues, extraordinary health issues, and assistance during expansion experiences. It's not only for expansion experiences. But I find that people often reach the point of feeling that they need more from their medical support system because of the physical and emotional pressure that expansion experiences place on them. Expansion experiences have traditionally been relegated to spirituality, and many feel that only those who are "spiritually evolved" have expansion experiences. Well, this simply isn't true. We all have expansion experiences. Any time we learn something new, that's expansion. Any time we experience something new, that, too, is expansion. Whatever is new to us must be received and processed accurately in order for the experience to be useful.

I have said that a good sign a person needs MAP is when he has a deep sense that he needs more medical support than is presently available to him. Many feel the need for additional help when struggling with especially challenging expansion experiences because, as a rule, traditional and alternative medical systems prevalent today do not accept or understand that the human body plays an essential role during expansion. They don't understand or accept how the body functions at these times or what help we need if we are not functioning well. The next session from Lorpuris will be helpful to those of you who recognize that you have been backed into a corner because of difficulties arising from expansion.

In explaining to me the role of the body in expansion, Lorpuris also gave a good explanation of how we operate as body/soul life systems on our planet. I think this will be helpful, in general, in understanding why we would feel the need for new medical assistance.

## *LORPURIS: HOW WE PHYSICALLY SUPPORT EXPANSION*

*An expanded experience does not by definition mean it to be nonphysical or beyond five-senses form. It simply implies that the experience is beyond that which the person has experienced prior to that time—thus, the sense of expansion. We have said to you that the band of form is quite complex, and this is true. It includes all that a person can potentially experience while participating within any given level of form such as Earth.*

*While participating within a level of form such as Earth, all reality adheres to the universal law of horizontal compatibility. Consequently, what is expressed within the Earth level is "of form" whether it be discernible to the naked eye or not. The limitation regarding form arises when an individual defines form strictly from the perspective of the five senses. Nature, for example, does not distinguish between the tree as seen by the naked eye and the nature spirit of the tree that is not seen. To nature, both are fully "of form" and, therefore, have impact on and respond to one another within the laws of form.*

*Now, the laws of form are much broader than what is encompassed when one thinks of the five-senses sensory system. In fact, an expanded experience is simply learning or allowing the sensory system, as most individuals know it, to operate in a fuller capacity.*

*The problem is that individuals see the five-senses system as the one and only sensory system, and anything beyond or outside this base functioning as being something entirely different. In fact, they are both functions of the same system.*

*When a child is born into the Earth level, its sensory system is quite sensitive and expanded. It is, after all, just moving from a state of being prior to birth in which the sensory system naturally functions in a broader state. If left on its own, the child would continue to develop its sensory system from the point of this broader perspective. And what one might call "expanded experiences" would be the norm. Societal preconceptions are what encourage the child to limit the sensory scope, and the development of the sensory system throughout childhood then takes place from this more limited perspective. Along with this, the limited definition of the sensory system and its scope of discernment becomes the rule of thumb by which to judge experience.*

*Now, if the sensory system is capable of naturally operating in a much broader scope than most individuals can at present imagine, it follows that the physical body must respond to and support that operation. The sensory system itself is a part of that overall body response and support system. Everything works as a team, ideally. Consequently, one cannot have what is known as an expanded experience without the sensory system and the physical body system as a whole responding to and attempting to support it. So, one may see a meditative state as an expanded experience, but, in fact, it is a broader use of the sensory system and draws appropriate response and support from within the physical body itself. Just as one cannot move a finger or toe without the entire body's muscular and skeletal systems responding, one cannot shift from one state of mind to another without a similar physical response and shift.*

*There is a saying many on the Earth level use: "If you don't use it, you lose it." Normally, this refers to muscle and body tone. When a child limits the scope of operation within the sensory system, the complementary scope of physical response and support is no longer needed or utilized. In those areas, a person stiffens and atrophies. Then, later on, when the individual is an adult and consciously chooses to reactivate the sensory system in a broader way, the physical body no longer "knows" how to respond and support that expansion. The person will experience nothing, no matter how much willpower he musters, or the experience will be partially perceived and most likely distorted, as well.*

*Let's address the body system itself and what happens when the sensory system responds to an experience. Any experience initially strikes the human body through the electrical system. This occurs whether the experience is easily perceived or not. The initial receptor of experience is not the brain or the senses but the electrical system. The impact immediately, almost simultaneously, shifts and translates into the nervous system and routes itself throughout the nervous system appropriately as it begins its identification and experience process. This includes activating the sensory system in an appropriate manner. (All this occurs within a split second.) The point to remember is that the initial level of impact is electrical, followed by an impact on the nervous system. If the experience is within the individual's perceived notion of "acceptable," this usually means that the person knows how to perceive the experience on all levels operating within the physical body.*

*Two things can occur if the individual doesn't know what to do with the experience. Either the body doesn't know how to respond and support the experience and is in need of assistance, or the experience itself is so beyond the person's operating scope of reality that it takes on an intensification that literally overwhelms the body and requires of it a level of operation well beyond its present range of capability.*

*In the latter case, the person must have a good foundation for such a stretch, or else he risks damaging himself physically. You would not want a person who is not capable of walking a half-mile to suddenly be forced to run three miles. But you could expect someone who easily runs three miles could tackle a seven-mile run without sustaining damage. It's a challenge, but it is not beyond the scope of possibility, and most likely not dangerous. However, the body used to the exertion of the three-mile run would have a challenge with responding well to the longer run, and it could result in soreness and discomfort until the body learns to support the longer run.*

*Addressing the case of your 1982 expansion, Machaelle: You had the foundation for the challenge. You could run the three miles with ease and grace. This we were sure of. The question was how you were going to process the intensity of the new input. All that occurred was initially received within the electrical system and then shifted into the nervous system. In some ways, you responded physically much more quickly than we anticipated. In other instances, the experience overwhelmed your system and assistance was needed. Note in the work done on you by the chiropractor that she maintained close proximity to the electrical and nervous systems by concentrating her work on the spine, sacrum and cranials.*

*Let me sum up the relationship of the cranial/spine/sacrum with the expanded experience. The experience is received electrically, shifted to the nervous system for sorting and identification, and, at this point, the physical body systems move to support what is being identified. If the body cannot adequately shift, the electrical system will overload or break, and the corresponding vertebrae, sacrum or cranials will most likely react by misaligning. Hence you have the sensation of trying to catch six balls all at once while only being able to catch four.*

## A Special Note About the Cranials

*An expanded experience carries with it an intensity that registers through the electrical system, moves into the nervous system, and continues its impact into the cerebrospinal fluid. The brain is impacted by both the nervous system activity and the CSF (cerebrospinal fluid) pulse response to the impact. The cranial plates must respond accordingly to accommodate this two-pronged impact. The range of plate movement will be affected. If the cranials have lost their knowledge of how to move within this new range or if they are three-milers stretching for the seven-mile run, they run the risk of jamming or misaligning. This is when so much of the head pain associated with expanded experience comes up. Cranial adjustments may be necessary over a period of time in order to allow time for the plates to properly adjust to and move in a more expanded range. One may receive these adjustments either from a physician such as a chiropractor or from MAP.*

*Just as the leg muscles need to adjust to the seven-mile run, the cranials need time to adjust to expansion. Because of the close working proximity with the electrical and nervous systems, the cranials must be considered one of the primary areas for assistance during times of expansion. In a relatively short period of time, the cranials, as well as the rest of the physical body system, will learn how to operate within the expanded range of experience with ease, accuracy and efficiency.*

*Chapter 3*

# *How to Work with MAP*

READ THROUGH THIS CHAPTER in its entirety before doing your first MAP session. It will give you a good foundation. There are quick-reference steps in Chapter 8 that you can use when doing a session.

## THE FIRST SESSION: UPDATED

Lie down. Get comfortable. You will need to lie on your back and remain in that position during the entire session, which lasts one hour. *Also, while lying down, do not cross your legs or your hands and arms over your body.* NOTE: If you have to do or get something during the session that requires that you cross your arms over your body, that's fine. When you're finished, just remember to put your arms back along your sides. Also, you might wish to cover yourself with a blanket, even a thin blanket in the summer. Besides keeping you warm, it may make you feel more secure. If you have back pain or are having trouble getting comfortable, try placing a pillow under your knees. If sitting in a comfortable chair makes it easier for you to remain alert and relaxed, then do it. In short, do what you need to do in order to remain alert and be comfortable.

By the way, the MAP team does not care if you are wearing clothes—or, in other words, they don't require that you get naked! You can wear a belt, polyester, naturally dyed garments or unnaturally dyed garments. What you are wearing is not an issue to the MAP teams. The only criteria is that you are comfortable.

1 Open the MAP coning. (Relax. Keep reading. "Coning" gets explained.) The MAP coning:

- Overlighting Deva of Healing
- Pan
- White Brotherhood Medical Unit
- Your higher self

To open this coning, state (aloud or to yourself): *I would like to open a MAP coning. I would like to be connected with the following members:*

- *the Overlighting Deva of Healing,*
  Wait ten seconds for the connection.
- *Pan,*
  Wait ten seconds.
- *the White Brotherhood Medical Unit,*
  Wait ten seconds.
- *my higher self.*
  Wait ten seconds.

Wait another ten to fifteen seconds to adjust to the coning.

The MAP coning is now open and you are ready to begin. It's that simple. It is not important if you did not have any sensations as the coning was activated. Your sensations or lack of sensations will not affect the quality of the coning in any way. What is important is that you be the one to call the coning into activation.

● ABOUT CONINGS. Since the 1990 publication of *MAP,* people have expressed interest in knowing more about a coning—what it is, what it does and how it works. You don't have to understand a coning in order to work with MAP. All you have to do is go through step 1 and the coning automatically opens. Then you can proceed with the session. If you want to know more about conings, turn to Appendix A. If this coning business doesn't interest you right now, just go on to step 2.

2 THE SCANNING. The first session will be for scanning purposes only. This is the one session when you need not talk to your team if you don't wish. The purpose of this session is to key you into their level, identify your various energy patterns, lock in your life systems on all PEMS levels, and get the appropriate medical team identified and working with you. This team will work with you during all your MAP sessions. Occasionally, when the situation calls for it, another member of the medical unit will join your team to lend expertise for a special situation. In these instances, the team will expand on its own to include whoever is necessary. You do not have to do anything special for this to occur. Your primary team will be those who work with you during all your sessions.

*The scanning session will last one hour.* You may feel gentle shifts and energy flowing throughout your body during this session. Or you may even feel like you are floating or moving. You also may feel absolutely nothing. Don't worry about this. The work is going on. You might want to set a timer or alarm for one hour when you begin the session so that if you should drift or fall asleep, you'll know when the session is over and when to go on to step 3.

3 YOUR CODE. At the end of the hour, request that you be given your code—a symbol, word, or sensation that you can use to identify your team. Whatever pops into your mind next will be it. Don't discount what happens once you request the code. When opening a coning for any future MAP sessions, add this identification (visualize or speak it) when you call the White Brotherhood Medical Unit into the coning. This will link you more efficiently with your team. Another way of saying this is: The code is the "extension number" you will use when connecting with your MAP team. It allows you to bypass the White Brotherhood's "main switchboard." It might be good to write or draw your symbol right after this first session just to make sure you recall it accurately later on.

Many have gotten nervous when they get to this part of the process because they feel they won't be able to discern their team identification or code. In fact, some use this as an excuse not to do MAP. Well, all I can say is that you've got to try this to believe it. Many people who swore they could never be "sensitive" enough to get their code have gathered in their courage and asked the question. Lo and behold, up pops their code. They hear a word or a phrase, or they visualize a scene, or suddenly recall a special scene from their past, or see colors, or hear sounds, or feel a strong, clear sensation. Whatever it is, that's their team identification.

Your team identification can be fun. They can sound like something out of a CIA code book: Torch, Lancer, Deep Rest, NIMO, Bunny-Love, Crystal Dove, or, my personal favorite, I Gotta Pee.... Other people get visual symbols: the peace symbol, trees, a specific flower, clasped hands, the sun, shafts of light.... And still others see one or more colors. When they open the coning, they identify their team by visualizing or looking at a specific color or pattern of colors.

These identifiers don't have to be wrought with deep esoteric meaning; they just have to be something that you and your team agree upon. And they're not secret. You don't compromise MAP or your team in any way if you share what your code is with others. And no one else can use your code. Someone else may have a code name that is similar, even the same as yours, but when that code is linked with you (i.e., *your* energy field), as it is when you are opening a MAP coning, it becomes unique to you, and you automatically connect with your team.

Also, I have heard from some folks who, after working with MAP for a while, wanted to change their identifying code or symbol. Sometimes they sense the name should be changed, or they feel that their team now has permanent new members. You can either request a new code from your team or suggest one yourself. What's important is that your team is very clear about the new identification. Or, you'll be in a session, not sensing that any change is needed, when a new code suddenly pops into mind. However the new code is derived, describe it fully to the team during that MAP session. Most likely, they will either flash the new symbol or "sound" the new code back to you to indicate their code for you has now changed. Or you can kinesiology test that it is acceptable with the team.

- If you don't hear or sense a code during this first session, relax. You can continue with MAP without a code. For future sessions, just continue to set up the coning as you did for this scanning session. You will then be connected with your team. It's like you call into the main switchboard and then your call gets transferred to the right party. As mentioned above, using the symbol makes this process more efficient. But not using a symbol doesn't prevent your having a MAP session. Eventually, you will "receive" the code.

4 Close the coning. At the end of the hour, close the coning. You do this by focusing on each member of the coning separately, thanking that member and stating that you would like to be disconnected from:

- Your higher self
- Your White Brotherhood Medical Team
- Pan
- Overlighting Deva of Healing

Wait ten to fifteen seconds for the dismantling to occur. A coning closes as easily as it opens. You need do nothing fancy.

If you are using Perelandra's ETS Plus, take one dropperful (ten to twelve drops) right after you close the coning. ETS Plus will help stabilize you after your first experience in a MAP coning. However, if you are not using ETS Plus, you'll be fine. Just spend a few moments quietly before going on about your day. Bouncing out of a MAP session without taking ETS Plus could feel like a jolt. (See Appendix C for information on ETS Plus.)

Wait twenty-four hours before opening the next session. The body needs twenty-four hours to adjust to the impact of the coning and the expansion of working with the White Brotherhood team. Once you have waited the twenty-four hours and you have done your first regular session, you need not wait twenty-four hours again before opening MAP. If you are sick, you may wish to open MAP daily for assistance as you move through the illness.

## REGULAR MAP SESSIONS: UPDATED

If you use ETS Plus, place the bottle within easy reach. If you do not use this or have never heard of it, I highly recommend that you investigate it and consider adding ETS Plus to your health program. Also, although optional, the MAP teams now prefer you to use ETS Plus. Prior to its development, it was recommended that you test flower essences during MAP sessions. With the development of ETS Plus, this part of MAP has gotten a lot easier. Now there is no testing involved. All you do is take a dose of ETS Plus (ten to twelve drops) where indicated. It is used in conjunction with the MAP sessions to stabilize us after the session and assist in our integrating the work the MAP team has done. There are times when the work will take, if left on its own, twenty-four hours to shift into and complete its impact on the physical body. ETS Plus makes these shifts efficient, effortless and complete within a two-hour period at the most. I have included information on ETS Plus in Appendix C. *But again, if you do not have ETS Plus, this does not stop you from participating fully in MAP.*

Lie down on your back or sit. Get comfortable. Cover yourself with a blanket if you wish.

1 OPEN THE MAP CONING. Wait ten seconds after each connection.

- Overlighting Deva of Healing
- Pan
- Your White Brotherhood Medical Team
  Visualize your team's symbol or say the code word.
- Your higher self

Wait ten to fifteen seconds after activating the full coning so that your body can stabilize itself within the coning and with the team.

2 Take ETS Plus. Take one dose (ten to twelve drops) of ETS Plus. If you are not using ETS Plus, skip this step.

3 Focus your attention on the session and your team. If you can't feel or sense your team, just keep your focus on the session. Describe as fully as you can how you are feeling. This includes how you feel physically, emotionally, mentally and spiritually. Relax about what you are not able to articulate. You get better with practice. *(Remember: This step is crucial for indicating your personal timing and rhythm. Your team will never alter or bypass your timing and rhythm. What you can articulate, you are ready to address.)*

- Symptoms. This is where people begin to feel like hypochondriacs or that they are pestering their team with "silly little things" that aren't really a problem.

Let me say something about symptoms that might help get you over this hurdle. Symptoms create a crucial, active communication between you and your body when you are not functioning in balance. They become an effective tool when we are working with a MAP team that understands the full ramification of each symptom and knows what to do with them.

In the medical world, symptoms are used for achieving an overall definition or label from which a doctor can choose a prescribed course of action, which is then superimposed onto the symptoms.

With MAP, symptoms are important tools for determining complexity, degree, rhythm and timing.

When describing symptoms to your team, be precise—or as precise as you can be. Don't just say you feel emotional when you could break it down by saying you feel teary eyed, vulnerable and easily irritated when people say certain things to you. (Then describe those things.) Don't just say you have a headache when you could be more specific by saying you have pain and pressure in the upper right side of your left eye and across the middle of your forehead. And learn the differences between an ache, a pain and a shooting pain.

Remember, symptoms are the communication between you and your body. By accurately describing them to your MAP team, they become the communication between you and your team, as well. The symptoms you are able to perceive and how accurately you are able to describe them tells your team precisely what you are ready to work on.

As I've said, your team isn't stupid. They know what your imbalances are. By describing how you are feeling to your team, you are telling them which of the imbalances you are ready to work with.

CAUTION: Some people have tried to get around this issue of talking to their team about symptoms by just giving the team a blanket invitation to work on everything—now. This is foolhardy, and your team will not accept the invitation. It would be risky to your health and well-being if you were moved from an imbalanced state to one of balance all at one time.

Also, many people diagnose their own symptoms. They're doing exactly what doctors do. I must admit that in a lot of cases, their guess is as good as the doctor's. They look at the collection of symptoms, then figure out what illness or disease these symptoms best describe. But I recommend that, when working with MAP, you do not self-diagnose. Just describe the symptoms. For example, don't say, "I have shingles." You might not have shingles, but apparently you know what constitutes shingles. Your label could get in the way of what is really going on with you, and although your team already knows you don't have shingles, what's important in this situation is what you think you have. You may have unwittingly created a block that has complicated your true illness, which can't be eliminated until you discard the self-diagnosis.

4 Allow forty minutes for the session to be completed. If you feel uncomfortable during the session, tell your team what you are feeling (this includes physical and emotional discomfort), and then relax and trust that at the end, whatever adjustments and shifts that were making you uncomfortable will have been completed.

● Optional—ETS plus during a session. If ETS Plus is available, take one dose at the onset of discomfort. The team will wait while you take this, then resume the session. Also, if you should get an intuitive hit to take ETS Plus, either check with your team and ask if they want you to take a dose (if you can directly communicate with them), or assume your intuition is correct and take the dose. However, before taking ETS Plus, tell your team you feel the need to do so. They will hold up their work while you do this. If your intuition was wrong, don't worry. ETS Plus will do no harm. It's certainly worth checking out, and your team does not mind if you do so.

● Moving around. It's important that you move around as little as possible during a session, so have the bottle of ETS

Plus beside you during the session. Also, if you change your position or need to go to the bathroom during a session, tell your team to hold it a minute, do what is needed as quickly as possible, lie down again and return to the session.

Sometimes their work will make you feel like you want to curl up in a fetal position. Don't do it. Just remain on your back and tell your team about this urge. Shortly the team will have moved you through the process so that you will no longer feel the need to curl up.

● TALKING/FEEDBACK DURING A SESSION. Don't be afraid to talk to your team during a session. It is especially helpful if you give them a running commentary of what sensations you are feeling, if any, so they can read on the spot how you are processing the work they are doing. If you suddenly feel pain, let them know where it is and how intense it is. Your body is working hard on all of its levels to make shifts and changes. Sometimes, something gets a little "hung up" in the process. That's why your feedback is so important. (They are also open to hearing any good jokes you might have as they work.)

Some people have said they feel odd talking to their team. After all, no one but you is visible in the room. They fear that anyone overhearing them may think they're crazy. It is helpful to speak out loud. Your team doesn't care; they can "hear" you if you say it out loud or silently. But it is helpful to *you.* When we speak out loud, it is easier—much easier—to maintain our focus on what we're saying. This is important if we are a little tired going into a session and intend to stay awake. So, I recommend that you say it out loud—but, you don't have to shout it! Just say it softly. Make sure you can hear yourself while, at the same time, no one in the next room can hear you.

5 CLOSE THE CONING. At the end of forty minutes (add a few minutes for opening the coning, disruptions, or bathroom time-outs you may have taken during the session), thank your team and close the session by dismantling the coning.

Dismantling the coning is as easy as activating it. State (aloud or to yourself): *I'd like to close the coning. I'd like to disconnect from:*

- *my higher self,*
- *my White Brotherhood Medical Team,*
- *Pan,*
- *the Overlighting Deva of Healing.*

Wait ten to fifteen seconds for the dismantling to occur. You may wish to spend an extra few minutes quietly before continuing with your day.

6 OPTIONAL. Take ETS Plus to stabilize the session. For this, you will need to take *three doses* of ETS Plus. Take the first dose immediately after closing down the coning. Wait five minutes, then take the second dose. Wait five more minutes and take the final dose.

## MAP Session Schedule

● IF YOU HAVE NO SERIOUS ILLNESS, DISEASE OR INJURY. The following schedule is how the team would like to work with you for the first five months. This schedule applies to those of you who can communicate directly with your team and those of you who cannot. After working with many thousands of people in MAP since 1990, the teams prefer this beginning schedule for those of you who do not already have a serious illness, disease or injury.

- The beginning schedule.
  - First month—twice weekly
  - Second through fourth months—once weekly
  - Fifth month and on—monthly
    (for balancing and general maintenance)
  - During times of difficulty, illness, or while going through periods of challenging expansion—twice weekly. If you sense more is needed: three or four times weekly.

After five months, the teams recommend that sessions be held monthly for balancing and general maintenance. However, if a specific difficulty, illness, or injury should arise during or after this five-month period, have MAP sessions twice weekly while going through these periods. If you sense more is needed to get you through the rough time, have sessions three to four times weekly. Once you are through this period, go back to where you were in the rhythm before the problem arose.

Once you can communicate with your team, either through kinesiology or intuitive input, after the five-month beginning schedule, you can ask for specific guidelines for the schedule that are geared to your personal needs. Or you can just remain on the monthly schedule until a specific need arises. Then have MAP sessions two, three, or four times weekly, depending on what you sense is needed.

- For those entering MAP with serious illness, injury or disease.

The MAP teams request the following schedule:

- First month—twice weekly
- Second through fifth month—once weekly

- Continue on the weekly schedule until you have moved through the illness, injury or disease.

After the fifth month, assuming you can communicate with your team, you may ask for specific guidelines for the schedule that are geared to your needs. If you cannot get this information, assume you are to stay on the weekly schedule if you are still moving through the illness, injury or disease.

Once you have completed the fifth month and you have completely moved through the serious problem, have MAP sessions twice a month for the next two months. After this, have a session monthly for balancing and general maintenance.

During times of difficulty, illness, or while going through challenging periods of expansion, go back to having sessions twice weekly. If you sense more is needed, have them three or four times weekly.

### Finding the Time to Do MAP

You've just gotten depressed because you don't know how in the world you are going to keep up with this schedule. Many people who have started MAP have faced this problem. A number of mothers of small children have told me that they actually get someone to babysit the kids during their MAP sessions. Others have said they play mind tricks on themselves—and they work! They say they pretend the MAP sessions are a class, or a doctor's appointment, or a racquetball game, or a meeting—something that requires them to literally carve out the time and create the schedule for it. To just have something to do at home doesn't give them enough of a reason to make the time. So they pretend it is one of those things that would normally force them to make the time. This shifts their attitude. Just by looking at the MAP schedule from a different perspective gives them what they need to adjust their lives in order to accommodate a session. There wouldn't be a question about working to accommodate an important meeting or class. They could do it. The mind game allows them to transfer that ability and apply it to MAP. If you're overwhelmed by this schedule thing, you might try this trick.

Of course, no amount of mind games or tricks will get you to actually schedule MAP if you really don't wish to do this kind of work. If you find you are becoming surprisingly creative about ways you can prevent yourself from having sessions, take the hint. You probably don't want to do this now. Put the book aside. At some point you will pick it up, read it again and find, much to your surprise, that you have no trouble scheduling those MAP sessions.

## You Can't Decide If You Want to Work with MAP

When you are deciding if you would like to participate in the program, I suggest that you make a five-month commitment to MAP—and then decide after the five months if you want to continue participating in the program. There are many things I can say about MAP and my experiences with it. But, to be honest, I can't adequately express to you in words how different and phenomenal this program is. You have to experience it for yourself. And, to appreciate what the program can do for you, you have to experience it for more than one or two sessions. After five months, you will have gone through all of the beginning schedule and established yourself in the once-a-month rhythm. I feel at that point you will be able to make a good decision. And, by that time, you will see that you really can integrate MAP into your life without causing a major upheaval to your schedule.

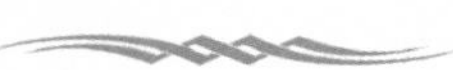

*Chapter 4*

# *Working with MAP and What Happens in a Session*

I HAVE WORKED WITH MAP personally and as part of the research and development at Perelandra since the summer of 1984. And I have gone through many different schedules with my team ranging from daily sessions to once a week or every three days. I have always allowed them to set a suggested pace, feeling that I would receive more from MAP both personally and as a researcher if I listened to my team. The scheduling for personal sessions did not correspond with specific physical or emotional "rough periods" when one might expect an increased need for MAP. Instead, they suggested an increase in sessions when my life became generally intense and it was imperative that my balance be maintained throughout.

What I would like to relate to you now are not only some of my experiences, but also suggestions based on others' experiences and work around MAP.

● HERE'S MY FIRST SUGGESTION. Read this chapter frequently as you develop your working relationship with MAP. It has a lot of helpful information in it—too much to absorb in one reading. People have asked me a lot of questions about MAP over the years, and I find that ninety percent of those questions were already answered in this chapter. With the third edition, there is even more information. So, consider this chapter your ongoing support and good friend.

## THE SESSIONS ARE ALWAYS DIFFERENT

I can never count on a session to be one way or another, even after all this time. When I think something is happening in my life that warrants a difficult session, I may get a gentle, easy one. I often have tough sessions when I least expect them. If I enter a session with a complaint about my right shoulder being stiff, I may feel them working on my left foot throughout the session. After the session, my right shoulder feels fine.

● THE SOFT SESSIONS. Sometimes, during the easy sessions I feel absolutely nothing. I know I am connected with my team and we may be "chatting" back and forth, but I can't feel them working on me. (I have accused them of gold-bricking!) At other times, I will feel my body gently move. I even feel that I'm being turned over or that I'm floating. Of course, when I look at myself, I'm still on the bed. But had I not opened my eyes, I would never have guessed that I had not physically moved. Sometimes I feel "electrical currents" flowing throughout my body or through part of my body. Sometimes I feel tingling sensations. All these things are quite pleasant.

● TOUGH SESSIONS. During the tough sessions, I feel pain. Sometimes—but not often—it's difficult pain. Usually the pain centers around emotional releases, and I have learned that emotional pain is truly as physically tangible as physical pain.

When the pain comes, I tell my team. Then I ask if I should take ETS Plus. Sometimes they say yes, sometimes they say it's not necessary. (If you can't "hear," this is where kinesiology testing comes in handy.) As intense as the pain may get, my team has *always* brought me full circle by the end of the session and the pain is no longer present. I have never left a session still having the pain. One of my suggestions to you, one I practice constantly, is to tell your team when pain occurs, how intense it is, where it is located and when the intensity either increases or decreases.

● BUBBLES. I have sometimes had a fun reaction when I was dealing with emotions in a session—the sensation that little "champagne bubbles" of energy float up through my chest and just pop out. This often makes me laugh.

● BREATHING. Sometimes I will be "bopping along" in my session, and all of a sudden, I will start deep breathing spontaneously and that will go on for some minutes. And then just as suddenly, I'll stop breathing deeply. During these times, I go with the impulses.

● CRYING. At other times, I cry. The odd thing is that it seems as if my team has hit a "cry button," and I just start crying. Sometimes I feel the specifics of the emotion, sometimes not. Sometimes insights surface, sometimes not. I also have had insights after the session when I was just going about my day again. Something comes to mind out of the blue, and everything from the session falls into place.

● POST-SESSION. Most of the time after a session, I feel fine. I have never been "left hanging" by my team. They seem to work in a rhythm that completes itself within the context of a single session. Sometimes I feel tired after a session, but a nap or a night's sleep takes care of that. Also, I usually feel vulnerable about the session itself, and I choose not to talk to anyone about the specifics. I feel close to my team and focus our work solely with them. But I've heard from others that they like to talk about their sessions. Their problem is finding someone to talk to. It helps them integrate the sessions.

● Delayed reactions. A handful of times over these past years, I have been absolutely fine after a session, and then the next day I take on a sudden, unexplainable pain that seems to come from nowhere. I have learned that at these times my body's adjustment to the work done has hit a glitch. I will take a dose of ETS Plus right away, then, as soon as I can, I will open a MAP session and tell them what is going on. Every time they have taken care of the problem.

Some have said that when this happens, and they only have a little time, they will quickly open a MAP coning and tell their team what is going on and that they can only give the team fifteen minutes. The team works fifteen minutes to take care of the problem. At the end of the session, the person takes a dose of ETS Plus. Then, within the next twenty-four hours, they will have a regular forty-minute session in order for the team to complete their work.

● Accidents. Being a part-time klutz, I am sometimes prone to an accident or two. I take ETS Plus immediately after *any* accident—minor or major. Then I open a MAP session and tell them what I have done to myself—this time. They have neutralized wasp stings, completely eliminated a black eye

(I hit my eye on a towel hook and it was well on its way to being a nasty black eye in about ten minutes), and worked me through a severely sprained ankle to the point that I was walking without a limp or pain in two days. They are also whizbangs at getting rid of sinus headaches.

● ASKING USELESS QUESTIONS. I don't ask my team a lot of questions about what they are doing. I know there are some people who are using MAP and just need to know *everything.* Oftentimes these people are not yet capable of communicating directly with their team and become frustrated about not knowing exactly what is going on. Quite frankly, I don't want to know all the nuts and bolts about what my team is doing. I sense that they are working in ways that I, at best, would barely understand. Instead, I focus on how I am reacting and responding to their work—and on the results of MAP. This way, I learn more about myself, recognize what I am experiencing from MAP, and am more capable of giving my team the feedback they need about how I am functioning. I let my MAP team do their job and I do mine.

● FALLING ASLEEP IN SESSION. When I first talked about MAP at a workshop, I cautioned people not to open a session if they are tired and likely to fall asleep. I still say this, but based on the letters I got back, I need to modify it a little. It is important that, whenever possible, you not come into a session in such an exhausted state that you conk out in the first five minutes. However, just about everyone who was working with MAP reported that they often fell asleep in the sessions no matter what they did. I asked Lorpuris about this, and he said that the team will put you in a sleep state at certain times when it is important for the work being done. Usually, an especially mentally active person who is getting "in the way" of the work will be put in a sleep state. When they need you to be alert, they will wake you up again. So, *your* responsibility will be to enter the MAP session when you can maintain alertness and can interact with your team. However, if you find you are going to sleep anyway, just relax about it. You've done your part by intending to be awake during the session.

● THE CANNON EFFECT. Sometimes you may feel you've just been fired out of a cannon! I think we have a wake-up button right next to that sleep button. The teams seem to use them both rather frequently. If you wake up with a jolt that frightens you or feels unpleasant, just tell your team and let them know you'd like something a little more gentle.

● WHEN THE FORTY MINUTES BEGIN. The forty-minute time for a session begins *after* the coning has been opened and you have taken the first dose of ETS Plus.

● SIMULTANEOUS AND NIGHT SESSIONS. If there are other people in your family who decide to work with MAP, your session schedules will not conflict with one another. You can all have your MAP sessions at the same time. MAP isn't a doctor's office where everyone has to wait his turn. However, if more than one MAP session is going on in the house simultaneously, make sure you are not in the same room. Each person needs to be in his own room.

Sometimes people wake up during the night and feel they need a session. You can have a session in bed next to your partner or spouse *if* you can get at least a three-foot clear space between you. Your team will have difficulty with the impact of another energy field from this person if he or she (or the dog) is too close. If you don't have enough clear space, you'll have to go into another room for the session.

- FAMILY ILLNESS. If the flu or any such illness is running through the family and you don't yet have it, nor do you want it, have frequent MAP sessions throughout the siege. Your team will help you maintain your balance and keep up your strength.

- MORE THAN PHYSICAL. Don't forget that MAP can work with more than physical issues. It is important for you to also bring up any emotional stress, mental pressures and spiritual conflicts. The PEMS levels are interrelated, and oftentimes your key to any one level hinges on your acknowledging and talking about the pains, pressures and conflicts going on at the other three levels.

- WHEN YOU NEED MORE THAN MAP. I have not needed surgery or broken any bones; consequently, I have not worked with MAP in these situations. But I have discussed this with Lorpuris, and I strongly suggest that you let common sense prevail and have needed surgery or broken bones set—and let MAP assist you during an emergency (see Chapter 6), surgery and recovery. In short, utilize the best medical practices possible for exceptional needs requiring quick physical attention. At the same time, look to MAP for assistance in any preparation you might require and the more complex areas of repair and healing resulting from the injury or surgery.

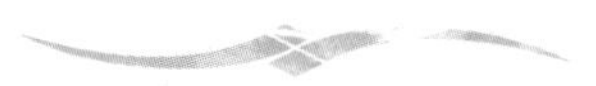

## HOW TO WORK BETTER WITH YOUR MAP TEAM

### Talking to Your Team

- Clearly define how you are feeling and list your current symptoms. Don't just focus on your physical glitches. Think about any emotional stress, mental strain, or spiritual conflict. An imbalance can show up on more than one level, and it is important to work with as much of the full problem as possible. Put all symptoms "on the table."

- Talk to your MAP team as if they know nothing about what is happening to you. Include everything that comes to mind as you are describing things to them.

- Give good follow-up. After a MAP session, be aware of any changes (good ones as well as the difficult ones) that happen to you on any level, even if the change doesn't seem to have any relationship to the things you talked about in the session. When you have your next session, tell your team about these changes. They will decide if the changes had anything to do with the work and what the changes mean in relationship to that work. The important thing for you is that you recognize that there have been changes.

  Hint: Keeping a list of the changes and referring to it during the next session can make life a lot easier for you.

- When you have no pressing symptoms and you are thinking about what to talk about in a MAP session, pick the issue that most stands out in your mind. Or, pick what jumps to mind first. But don't dump.

● DUMPING. I have written that whatever symptoms you have, tell your team. I'm not changing this. Whatever symptoms you feel before going into and during a session indicate the things you are ready to work with. However, believe it or not, there will be times when you will feel symptom-free. And you will have specific issues in mind that you would like to work on with MAP. Don't treat these issues like symptoms and throw every issue you can think of "on the table" in one session. You are going to overwhelm yourself.

Here's what you can do instead. List all the issues you'd like to work on with your team. Then, choose the most important issue to work on first, and gradually work your way down the list in future sessions. Better yet, ask your team which issue *they* recommend and get an intuitive hit or kinesiology test (if you can't hear their answer) to discern which issue should be worked on first. Once you have moved through this issue satisfactorily, review your list of issues and find out what you are to work on next. Continue doing this until there is nothing left on the list. (No need to feel you have to rush through your issues list. It'll keep you busy for years.)

If you overload a session by introducing too many issues, that can overload *you* as you try to comprehend all of the team's input. If you throw your team fifty balls, they may throw fifty balls back to you. The question is whether or not you are capable of catching that many all at once.

● YOU WILL BE CONSTANTLY IMPROVING and developing your ability to communicate with your team. A major key in working with MAP well is not what your team could say to you; it is what you say to your team. What you say indicates the speed and scope of change you wish to accomplish with your team. If you can't say it, they won't work on it. They assume that if you can't talk about it, it is not time to work on it.

A suggestion from my experience: I meet with my team often. It's not that I am in such bad shape—actually, I'm in terrific condition—but we meet to work out MAP-related issues, etc. One thing I've learned is that giving full and accurate input is an art form. It's like looking through a telescope that is constantly expanding to reveal more of the picture. When we focus on what we're seeing, we think we're seeing the whole picture. But the next time we look through the telescope, we discover there are entire areas—huge areas glaring out at us—that we were not aware of.

During one session, I asked my team to help me learn to observe my situation better and to give them better, quality input. They said to concentrate my efforts on improving the quality of my input to them—keep fine-tuning what I communicate. Over the following months, with the help of my team, I made dramatic changes in my ability to perceive a situation. Now, what I say to them is more comprehensive. For example, when I talk about something that is physically distressing, I am better able to pick up more of the nuances surrounding the distress. And I remember to add those subtle things on the other three levels that at one time I thought could never in a million years be related to the physical problem—but were. As a result, the MAP team is able to work with me in deeper, more effective ways. My movement with them has improved manyfold.

This input business is such a detailed, comprehensive art form that I don't see myself mastering it for a long time. It is a fascinating internal journey that develops personal discipline and life tools in ways that are simply unimaginable. I recommend it to all of you. Just ask your team to help you improve your perception and ability to communicate what you see, think and feel. Then, focus on giving your team the best input you can give. You'll see the changes. And have patience with yourself. Give yourself time to learn.

● INCLUDE THE POSITIVE. Surprise your MAP team. Tell them the good stuff that's going on in your life—and include any good insights you have had. By concentrating on the tough stuff, we are implying that only the tough stuff in our lives molds and moves us. This is nuts! So give the good stuff a hearing. (Does this sound like I'm standing on the sidelines madly cheering you on?!)

● FEELING STUCK. You've brought up a problem that you and your team have been working on. You feel like you've done everything but the problem remains. You feel like you've hit a wall and don't know what else to say or do. Well, you *have* hit a wall, but it's not with your team. It's a wall inside yourself. Ask your team to give you insight about what to do. The insight will help you move through or around the wall and you'll be on track again.

Better yet, do a MAP/Calibration around the fact that you have hit a wall either with your work with MAP in general or with a specific issue. (See Chapter 5 on MAP/Calibration.)

● HEARING/SEEING YOUR TEAM. I suggest that you relax about this. *Many* people don't get any kind of communication in a session. You don't need to hear or feel anything to participate in MAP. Your verification that something is really happening will be in the changes you feel around issues you've brought up in the sessions. Your whole focus will be on how you are responding to their work.

I know everyone would prefer to hear and see their teams. But whether one does depends on the range of function of their sensory system. It's as simple as that. Desire, deep concentration, worry and wishes won't make a difference. As I said, hearing and seeing the teams depends on our range of sensory function. When I am in a MAP session, I can hear my team clearly, but I can't see them. From talking about this issue in the workshops, I find out that a handful of people in the class can both hear and see. A larger number can experience one or the other, but not both. Equal in number to these two groups are those who can neither hear, see, nor sense their team. These people are always surprised to learn how many are in the same boat as they are. Many of these people say they feel their team communicates with them by giving them intuitive insights as they go about their normal daily schedule.

What has been made clear is that some people who start out sensing nothing gradually expand their sensory systems to where, six months to a year down the road, they can indeed hear and/or see their teams. And then there are most people who have exceptional success working with MAP and never hear or see their team.

● KINESIOLOGY IS THE BRIDGE TO YOUR TEAM if you can't hear them. As long as you know how to use kinesiology, you will be able to get answers to any of the questions you might have about your health and health practices. All you need to do is formulate the questions in a simple yes/no format. (See Appendix B for how to do kinesiology.)

Communication with your team will be more accurate and

have greater range if you use kinesiology instead of relying on intuition. It's tough to get clear, correct, precise and complex information through intuition unless you are well-disciplined in this area.

• IMPORTANT. Many people who have had trouble feeling a clear yes/no response with their kinesiology asked their teams to help them achieve the needed (and desired) clarity. They report that the kinesiology problems cleared up quickly and easily. So, let your team help you with your fears and difficulties as you develop this tool.

## The MAP Coning and Team

● CHANGING THE MAP CONING. A MAP coning is very precise, and it is set up as the MAP teams and nature wish. It is their program. It has been set up to give anyone who wishes quality health care in a perfectly safe environment. It was researched and developed for seven years prior to our offering the program to the public. Please consider this if you are toying with the idea of changing the makeup of the coning or how the program is set up. Some people have consciously worked in interlevel ways with souls prior to MAP. They feel that they must include these souls in the MAP coning. This is not true and it is also not helpful. MAP is a specialized coning designed and set up for comprehensive health care for those of us on the Earth level. It's not helpful to "load" others into the MAP coning who are not participating in the program. Anyone who should be a part of your medical team will automatically be included when the team is formed during the scanning session. If you would like to know if a soul you have already known and worked with is also part of your MAP team, just ask your team. They don't consider this secret information.

If, despite all that I've said, you feel compelled to alter the MAP coning or change any part of the program, always consult your team first—as a matter of courtesy, if for no other reason. Get their okay. And know that any approved changes in your coning or program are made just for you and are not to be passed on to others.

If you arbitrarily decide that you would like to set up the coning with different members or refer to the MAP-coning members by names that really do not apply to them, you will not have a MAP coning. Instead, you will have a coning comprised of those you have called in. And whatever happens while you have this coning activated will not be a MAP session. I am not saying that bad things will happen to you. I am only saying that when you arbitrarily change the composition of this coning, you no longer have a MAP coning. You may have a peaceful, even interesting session, but it will not be a MAP session. (For how to set up other conings, see Appendix A.)

• ADDING RELIGIOUS LEADERS. Some people feel more comfortable if they include Jesus Christ in their MAP coning. He is a member of the White Brotherhood and will be glad to join your coning. But He is not part of the medical teams and will not be working with you medically. He will be present in a supportive capacity.

• MAP TEAM GENDER MIX. Half of the MAP team originates from the White Brotherhood. (The other half is nature.) "Brotherhood," in this instance, means "all" as in "all life." It does not mean "men." Do not assume your team is made up solely of men. But, if you feel you do have a bunch of men—or a bunch of women!—and this makes you uncomfortable, say something to your team. Their feelings won't be hurt. They will adjust the makeup of your team appropriately.

● THE TEAMS OPERATE BEYOND TIME AND SPACE. There is no issue, as far as they are concerned, about your needing or wanting a session at 3 A.M. You are not waking them up and you are not pestering them. Have sessions at a time that is convenient to you.

In this same area, your team doesn't wake you up for a session. You will not be disturbed by them. They may not exist in time and space, but they are well aware of those dynamics—and that *we* exist in time and space.

● ABOUT YOUR HIGHER SELF. When I instruct you to connect with and disconnect from your higher self, I do not mean to imply that you haven't been connected all along. You cannot exist without a strong, functioning bond with your higher self! However, for MAP and other coning work, you temporarily expand the range of connection so that you can have *clear, conscious interaction* between your higher self and your conscious self. It takes a lot of physical energy to maintain this expanded connection. For your balance and well-being, it is important to readjust the connection back to your *normal range* once you have completed the work that required the special connection in the first place. If you don't do this (or you forget), you will experience an energy drain.

Some people have ignored my warnings about this. They want to be connected to their higher selves in this expanded range all the time. However, if they had been physically capable of maintaining such a connection indefinitely, they would not have had to expand the range in the first place. They would be automatically functioning in the more expanded range. It only takes a day or two to feel the effects of trying to maintain this connection. They feel run down, exhausted and sometimes lethargic. If you should ignore my warnings and find yourself in the same situation (and you wish to get out of it), just disconnect from your higher self as described when closing a coning. This will immediately adjust the connection to your normal day-to-day range. Then get some rest and eat a couple of high-protein meals. In a day or two you will be back to your old self—and glad for it!

## Problem Sessions

● Seeking instant perfection. Some people who are doing MAP have told me that they gave everything over to their teams. Basically they made a blanket statement at some point in their MAP development (usually right at the beginning) that the team was to do whatever was needed to make them "perfect." But then they were disappointed because not a whole lot was happening.

MAP doesn't accept that kind of blanket surrendering. You are creating a partnership with them and not surrendering yourself as a child to a parent. Plus, when *we* say "take it all and do everything" we don't necessarily realize what this implies. MAP requires that you consciously and knowingly request their assistance in specific areas. If there are areas in need of assistance that you don't understand or know about, the team will gently help bring these areas into your consciousness so that you can make appropriate decisions. How you proceed tells your team in what directions you'd like to go. Try to remember that your MAP team is extraordinarily expansive in what it knows and can do. Therefore, you must indicate to them *your* directions and pace so that they work with you specifically within the framework that *you* define.

● APPROPRIATE SESSION ENVIRONMENTS. Most of you would not arrange for a surgeon to do a biopsy on you while you are in your car driving to work. (Notice I hedged my bets and said "most.") You and the surgeon would prefer the work be done in an appropriate environment. The same is true with your MAP team. They don't want to work on you while you are driving to work. (By the way, I'm using this example because someone boasted to me that they actually did this.) Your MAP team doesn't ask for a lot. But they do insist that you be alone, alert for the session, and unoccupied with anything else during the session. If you open a session while in an inappropriate setting, the team will not work on you. They'll just wait quietly until you close the coning.

● MAP IS A MEDICAL PROGRAM. These teams will not make real estate or employment recommendations, they will not focus on how your business is doing, and they don't care about what your local city council is deciding. It is a *medical* program, and it deals only with your medical issues. If you like working with a coning, and you would like to set one up for a nonmedical area in your life, please do so. But don't bring it to MAP. (See Appendix A for setting up other conings.)

Nonmedical projects are called "soil-less gardens" and Perelandra has an entire program you can use for setting up a soil-less garden for any nonmedical project you wish. Many people work with soil-less gardens and report extraordinary successes. (For information, see our web site or current catalog.)

● MAP IS A MEDICAL PROGRAM FOR HUMANS—NOT ANIMALS. The team members are not veterinarians. They specialize in the human body. If you wish to assist an animal in a similar program, use the Nature Healing Coning for Animals. (See Chapter 11.) This was designed specifically for animals and is as effective for them as MAP is for us.

● ANIMALS IN YOUR SESSIONS. Animals absorb stressful human energy patterns. If you've ever had an argument with someone while your dog or cat was in the same room, and then watched the animal's behavior change right before your eyes, you know what I'm talking about. A lot of deep work goes on with you during a MAP session. Just because an animal wants to be near you while you are quietly sitting or lying down does not mean that animal wants or needs to experience your MAP session. And your team doesn't want to work with you while you have a cat plunked on your chest or lap. The two energy fields are going to commingle, and this isn't helpful for your team. Do you, your team and your animals a favor and don't include animals in your sessions.

● MAP JUNKIES. MAP is fantastic. There's no doubt about this. Most people who experience MAP say they have never experienced anything like it in their lives. But some people have gotten hooked on the program and have jumped off the deep end with it. They have sessions multiple times a day. And they insist that the sessions remain open for hours at a time.

MAP is a program that was designed to be integrated in a *balanced* manner into your life. It is not designed for taking over your life. The teams deal with a MAP junkie with terrific patience. They will work in a focused manner to help that person achieve a sense of appropriate balance in his life. At some point, the person will be hit with common sense and, hopefully, work with their team in a more balanced way. I say "hopefully" because sometimes the person will overreact and reject MAP altogether. They blame their "addiction" on MAP.

If you feel you might be a junkie and wish to achieve a more balanced relationship with MAP, just talk to your team about this. Describe your feelings about the program, how you feel when you are in a session, and how you feel when you are not in a session. Let them work with you on this issue.

## Comprehending What's Happening

You don't have to be able to hear your team talk to receive understanding about what is going on with you. MAP comprehension comes from insights and understanding that happen in various ways. Don't assume your team is going to write things down for you on golden tablets. The insights usually occur within the context of your everyday life. Often, you may be walking along a week or so after a session, thinking about absolutely nothing or humming some song when, all of a sudden, out of nowhere, you'll have an insight. It doesn't hit you hard. But suddenly a light goes on. It's a quiet thing. Also, pay close attention to your dreams. You may get a lot of insight and understanding this way, as well.

Comprehension often relies on new thinking. You may not be able to comprehend what's new with your old thinking. If you are working on a health issue (physical, emotional, mental, or spiritual) with MAP, this implies that you are having difficulty with that issue—otherwise, you wouldn't bother bringing it up. The resolution of many issues requires new thinking, new insights. The MAP team will "slip" these to you in unexpected ways. This catches you off guard so you won't mentally reject the insight or alter it and then fit it comfortably into your old thinking.

Don't be afraid to tell your team that you are totally at a loss about something. Actually, I say this to my team pretty often. It tends to be just the thing I need to admit that will then break up the logjam. I find that it's as good for us to articulate how much we don't know as it is how much we do know.

Also, don't assume you have to understand everything. You only have to understand what's relevant. Some things can occur in a session that are part of the issue being worked on but are not key to it. In order to understand the issue, you do not need to understand this one thing. Trust that your team will make sure you get the insight and information that is relevant to the issue—and let the rest float on by you.

● A REMINDER ABOUT REPORTING YOUR INSIGHTS. Once you have an insight, be sure you report it to your team in the next session. This way, your team knows you "got it," and while listening to you, they can tell how much of the insight you were able to grasp. This is how you communicate the pace and scope of your movement through issues. So, be clear and concise with your descriptions and understandings. (This is another reason why it's important to stay awake, if you can, during a MAP session. You really need to talk.)

Also, I pay attention to whatever pops into my head as I describe an insight to my team and include this in what I'm saying. Sometimes an event that occurred in my past will pop up and, as I describe it, certain emotions surface. The old event and the insight may not be related. But the emotions the old event activated may be crucial to understanding the insight.

### Reaction to Sessions

You had a MAP session, came out of it fine, and took ETS Plus. Then, sometime within the next twenty-four to thirty-six hours you began to feel unwell. You sense you are having a "reaction" to something that occurred during the session. You are scheduled to have another session next week. Here's what to do. Take a dose of ETS Plus right away. Then open a session as soon as possible and let them know exactly how you feel. When this happens to me, I usually feel like "something slipped" and I need to have the team "put it back into position." After this session, you'll be back on track. Before closing the session, ask if your schedule has changed. Don't assume they still want to see you in a week.

● IF YOU HAVE NO TIME FOR A SESSION. Have a quick session. Let's say you have fifteen minutes before you have to leave the house. (Or a fifteen-minute break at work, and you can have privacy. Bathrooms are good for this.) Open a session and let them know how you feel and that you only have fifteen minutes (or however long you have). Have the session and take one dose of ETS Plus, if you have it available. When you do a quick session, you must follow it up with a regular forty-minute session within twenty-four hours. After the follow-up regular session, ask if your schedule from your original session (the one before the quick session) has changed.

The following is from an article published in our newsletter, *Perelandra Voices.*

*I began doing MAP during Christmas vacation. It was difficult to return to work and put my energy in outer things. These sessions are, in some ways, hard work. My first day back at work, I got home beaten and frazzled after a long day. I was so exhausted—mentally, physically, emotionally—that I was unable to cope and in a state of panic and totally overwhelmed. I didn't have time to do a full MAP session. My husband was due home in twenty minutes. So I called a quick MAP session of twenty minutes (I didn't know if this was "legal," but I had to do something.) The first five minutes I sobbed hard, then felt sedated again. About halfway through, I felt a sudden intense electrical shock go through a joint of my ring finger—it jerked my arm off the bed and made me cry out. Then, nothing else. At the end of twenty minutes, I was in a totally different state. I was still a little tired, but I did all the things I needed to do that evening without strain, anxiety, or fatigue. On the contrary, I felt emotionally calm and peaceful. This may not sound like much to you, but it is a true miracle to me.*

E.R., Oregon

## Scaffold Sessions

To write about this effectively, I must lean on my personal background and my resulting experiences in this area.

When I was twelve years old, I became what is known today

as a throwaway child. This led to a number of years of difficult experiences. I'm being a little glib here because the details are not the issue right now. Suffice it to say that those early years, prior to being sent out on my own and after, were most unpleasant and challenging.

Part of my coming to terms with this time and these experiences was to process what happened, how I felt about it then and how I feel about it as an adult. As a result of this reflection, I reached a level of internal balance. I was happy and certainly quite functional. I did not feel as if those early years weighed me down at all.

Another way to look at the internal balance that I felt is to say that as I addressed and moved through each issue, a scaffolding was created inside me. Each issue became part of the scaffold. When I could feel internal balance, the scaffold was fully formed and served to give me a new supportive strength. I had taken what at one time was destructive to me, worked it over, turned it around, and created from these same experiences a scaffold of strength. I don't believe that this scaffold phenomenon is unique to me. On the contrary, I feel that this happens inside each of us as we address certain painful life issues. We can choose for our life experiences to create a scaffold of weakness and destructiveness, or we can take those same experiences, turn them around and create a strong, supportive scaffold with them.

For many years, my scaffold gave me a good, strong, workable balance. Then in 1982, I expanded my life in a way that required that I seek a new level of balance. One result of this is MAP. The heretofore perfectly fine scaffold had to be shifted to accommodate the new balance. That meant that it had to be dismantled. Each piece had to be either modified and placed differently, or released altogether. And sometimes, this can be tough.

This scaffold work is a real, physical dynamic. It is not some mental construct I've invented. We must physically, emotionally, mentally and spiritually shift in order to modify and reposition or release these scaffold pieces. From this, we create a new scaffold that strengthens and supports us on our new level in life.

MAP creates a safe environment for you. And every cell in your body knows this. So, where you might normally resist making these deep and challenging changes without MAP, you will most likely be inclined to actually say yes to them because of MAP. This program gives you a feeling of both support and safety. And there couldn't be a more appropriate environment for you to face these changes head on and make them.

An important point about scaffold sessions: You will not enter into this kind of session unless you are both ready and willing. Your team does not drag you kicking and screaming into a tough session. You may not consciously know what is ahead of you, but you have consciously put yourself in position for this, and your heart and soul have said yes. The teams do not trick you into a tough session. All they do is support you in every way as *you* prepare for and move through these sessions.

You might have some intense reactions in scaffold sessions when these pieces are being addressed, modified, repositioned, or released. You can experience intense physical pain, either generally throughout your body or localized in an area that is related to the scaffold piece being worked on. You may have a sudden and deep feeling of anguish descend on you, and you don't know what's causing it. You may feel the need to scream. Or the need to vomit. (My personal favorite.) You may feel unable to move or speak. And often, you will feel a strong desire to curl up in a fetal position. (It's important that you do not actually curl up. Remain in your usual session position.) ETS Plus can support you well through this process, so have a bottle close at hand.

I have never known beforehand when I am going to have a tough session. They just happen. When they have occurred, my team kept me in the session for ninety minutes. This allowed them the time to make sure the changes were complete and stabilized. I have never come out of a session feeling that I was left hanging. Each time I have had a scaffold session, I have come out of the session feeling a deep sense of peace.

In my twenty-three years working with MAP, I'd say I've had a total of fifteen sessions I would call tough. Most of them occurred in the early years. I haven't had any in a number of years. But I don't rule out the possibility of having tough sessions in the future. I have no fears about them. I know I'm perfectly safe.

Another thing: Most of the time I cannot identify what specific piece of my scaffold is being worked on. I can be having all kinds of reactions, but they're not connected with any piece of information that would give me insight as to what is occurring. I also don't ask for insight. If it's important for me, my team will make sure I get it. If it's not important—and most of the time it's not—I don't want to be bothered. As far as I am concerned, I'm ready to make the shift and I just want to get on with that process.

By the way, not all scaffold sessions are tough. Most of the pieces move into place quickly and effortlessly. As I said, tough sessions don't occur often. But when they do, they can be quite something.

● What to do if you should find yourself in a tough session. First of all, automatically assume you need to extend the session to last ninety minutes rather than forty minutes. Second, don't panic. You are in the best hands and you are fine. Tell the team everything you are feeling—every physical, emotional, mental and spiritual pain. Tell them when you want to curl up, when you feel so mentally restless you could scream, when you feel chilled or overheated. I also include when I'd like to punch out my team for this session I'm in. It gives them something to think about, and I feel better for having made the threat! All of this gives them feedback about how you are doing and where they need to shore you up. If you have to vomit or go to the bathroom, tell your team. They'll put everything on hold while you take care of business. The ninety minutes does not include a bathroom break, so you will need to add this to your session time.

After one of these sessions, you might want a nap and you might feel vulnerable. You will also feel peaceful. Later, if you have any discomfort resulting from the session, take ETS Plus and see your team as soon as possible.

### Frightening MAP Experiences

The MAP teams do not do things to scare you half to death. I've heard many refer to their teams as "gentle" and "loving" beyond belief. MAP teams do not throw things around the room or at you. They do not steal money from your wallet, or keep your body in perpetual sessions and refuse to "let go" even though you beg them to. They do not take over your life or tell you what to do or say. They do not wake you up every morning at some ungodly hour. In fact, they don't wake you up at all. Nor do they rip flowers out of your garden. These are all actual accusations people have made against their MAP teams. Here's some more of what they don't do: They don't automatically connect with you without permission, solve business problems, discourse on local government issues, heal animals, work on others without the other person's *conscious* permission, and they won't suggest that for the betterment of your soul you should become a tree.

This is not some intergalactic street gang you've teamed up with. They have the highest integrity. They will not work with you in harmful ways—and they will not harm you, period.

Now, if you have frightening experiences, MAP is not doing them to you. You are doing them to yourself. You are scared beyond words, and being in MAP isn't helping the situation. If you are having this experience, tell MAP immediately and take ETS Plus. If your fears and frightening experiences have not disappeared within one or two more sessions, *stop doing MAP altogether*—and right away. You are fighting yourself and you are not capable, in your present condition, of clearly discerning what is going on in a session. You are translating it in terrible, frightening ways. You need to do more personal balancing work around the causes of your fears to be able to perceive a session accurately before re-entering MAP.

People who have serious victimization, paranoid, or schizophrenic tendencies are especially vulnerable. Although MAP is perfectly capable of assisting people with these problems, the

MAP program itself can exacerbate their problems. In these instances, MAP is not for them. Good, qualified counseling or therapy is the way to go in these situations.

● HEARING VOICES. Another issue involves constantly hearing voices. MAP teams usually work quietly, unless you ask them something or are talking to them. They are not chatterboxes by any means. A couple of people have said that their teams talk all the time to them—within a session and outside a session. They say they have asked the teams to stop, but they won't. And they say that their teams are telling them to do odd things. One fellow was "told" to have an affair with his neighbor. Another was being "told" to fuse with and become one with the aforementioned tree, and once she did this, she would be able to serve the world in new and wondrous ways.

I hate to disappoint you folks out there, but MAP teams are actually quite reasonable in both what they talk about and how they say it. They really don't sound like a bunch of New Age freak-outs. Their demeanor is polite, kind, caring, respectful, supportive—and always professional.

What's happening with these people is that they are hearing themselves. MAP has gotten them both excited and scared, and they've fallen off into fantasy conversations that they attribute to MAP because the talks sound just like what they imagine a MAP team would say. And they think the teams are "saying" exactly what the person wants to hear.

Sometimes, these people are unhappy with their lives and yearn to do something "significant." The yearning becomes so great that it trips them over the edge, and they begin to hear voices telling them how great they are and what they need to do to help save the world. Again, they are hearing themselves.

HERE'S WHAT TO DO IN THIS SITUATION: Tell your team you're being hounded by voices. Also tell your team you plan not to take the voices seriously anymore. (And then don't take them seriously anymore! Don't do anything or say anything based on what these voices are saying. In short, render them powerless.) From that point on, your team will work with you without saying a word. They will also not communicate with you through kinesiology. Most likely, if you have been using kinesiology, you are not sure if you are controlling the testing. By the team maintaining silence in these two areas, you won't have the problem of trying to discern who is talking. If they need to get something across to you, they will do it in another way, but it won't be verbal. Then they will work with you to move you into a more balanced position where you will no longer hear any voices.

You won't be able to ask them about a session schedule because your team is no longer talking to you. So, plan to have weekly sessions until the voices disappear. Then have sessions twice a month for the next two months. After this, have sessions monthly.

● THERE IS A DIFFERENCE BETWEEN A TOUGH SCAFFOLD SESSION AND A FRIGHTENING EXPERIENCE. A scaffold session can be tough because of a strong reaction or response you are having as a result of the work being done. A frightening experience usually involves some perceived attack either by the team or some outside force. Because of the coning, no force outside the coning can disturb you in any way. You are fully protected.

## Trying to Control Your Team

Some people try to control or "corner" their MAP team. These people want something or need to make sure they are right about something. They usually attempt to control their team by how they ask the team questions. For example, if a person really wants to have MAP sessions three times a day, he will ask questions about his schedule that will ensure that the answer leaves open the possibility of super-frequent sessions. For example, rather than asking how often he should have sessions, he will ask if having sessions as often as he would like is okay. If he is discerning the answer through kinesiology, the answer will most likely be positive. It's okay. What the team is really saying is that it is okay, but it is not needed nor is it particularly useful. By the way the question is phrased, the person hasn't allowed for this kind of input from the team. In order to get full information, you may have to ask a series of questions. You ask the main question, then ask additional questions that allow for any modification or qualification of the main question. The way to continue the schedule questioning with your team would be to also ask if frequent sessions are *needed.* Now you've given your team a chance to say "okay, but not needed."

The team will not work on you in useless or harmful ways. The people who ask these kinds of limiting or controlling questions can open a MAP session as often as they like. But, most likely, the most significant issue the team will be working on is your addiction to MAP sessions.

When asking for information from your team, look at how you are phrasing the questions and see if you are presenting them in a manner that supports your own desires. In short, are you being honest in what you are asking. In this kind of situation, you are not controlling your team, you are controlling yourself. Your team knows exactly what you are trying to do. And, as I said, they will work with you to overcome this situation, but they will not participate in your efforts to control or manipulate them.

Another issue occurs when you wish to control the answer by asking your team a question and then supplying only the options or actions you desire to follow. For example, you have verified that your team is suggesting a change in diet. You can't hear them tell you the changes, so the only way to get the information is by using kinesiology. You test a list of things that are in your current diet. You are asking the question, "Do I eliminate this item?" That's all fine, except that you chose to leave a few things off your list—like the daily three martinis and pint of Ben and Jerry's Heath Bar Crunch ice cream. In this situation, MAP will answer you according to the best of the options you have given. However, it may not be the best option overall for you. When you give options, remember to add at the end of your list "none of the above." This allows your team to get across to you that you are going to have to expand your options if you want the best answer.

Keep questions short, clear, clean and honest. If you are using kinesiology, you will need to ask them in a simple yes/no format. The simplicity of this format is helpful in maintaining clarity whether we are using kinesiology or hearing our team directly—and simplicity makes it easier to spot our creative attempts at control. (To learn kinesiology, see Appendix B.)

## Session Aerobics and Sleep

● SESSION AEROBICS. I've written about not moving physically or crossing your limbs during the session. Let me qualify this. It's important that you remain physically quiet during a session. Don't toss and turn. Don't cross your arms over your chest and don't cross your legs. But sometimes you'll sense a specific movement—like a clear impulse to move in a specific manner. This probably is something your team wants you to do and may be related to an adjustment they are working on. Go with the motion. If you can hear your team, ask them if they'd like you to do the movement. If you are communicating through the use of kinesiology, ask the same question and test for the answer. If you do neither, but have a strong sense of a well-defined movement, go with your gut instinct, tell your team what you are about to do—and do it. These movements are not complicated. Nor do they last long. It's not as if you are going to do tough calisthenics for forty minutes. (And it does not include running to the store for a six-pack!)

● SLEEP. I'm repeating this in several places because it is such an issue with people. Go into the session wide awake. If you fall asleep during the session, don't worry about it. You have fulfilled your responsibility entering it awake, alert and capable of remaining that way. But if you do fall asleep, despite these efforts, it is most likely a reaction to the work your team is doing. Or, your team needs to "get you out of the way" mentally while they work. Intelligent, inquisitive people often conk out during their sessions. Most likely, they were too active mentally and were interfering with the work that was being done. (I haven't met anyone yet who hasn't fallen asleep in a MAP session—myself included.)

If you wake up and realize that the session was probably over two hours ago, or it's the next morning and you never closed the session, it's okay. Your team won't send you a bill for time and a half. Close the coning now, and take the three doses of ETS Plus. You haven't inconvenienced your team. Remember, they operate beyond time and space, so your clock is not an issue to anyone but you.

If you tend to go to sleep and need to make sure your session doesn't run over a certain time, set an alarm clock for yourself. Just make sure you are not cutting your forty-minute session short.

## Menopause and Gynecology

Menopause is a natural cycle and is therefore well understood by both nature and the White Brotherhood. It need not be a time of internal chaos because it is a change that (naturally) has its own unique order and organization. But it can feel chaotic if its order and organization (balance) is off. If you read the *Co-Creative Definitions* (Appendix E), you'll see that nature supplies all of reality's order, organization and life vitality.

As we women approach the menopause years (or *feel* we are entering that time), we can open a MAP/Calibration session and request that we be prepared for the changes so that we can enter the time in appropriate balance. (But, be prepared! This may require some lifestyle changes such as in your diet, exercise and drinking habits!) Once requesting the help of your team, ask if you are to have a MAP/Calibration *series* of sessions specifically for menopause preparation. If so, get that schedule. It may extend over months, even longer.

As we move through menopause, we can do MAP/Calibration often to maintain the unique balance that menopause requires. We can talk about all the changes as they occur, our reactions and perceptions. And we can talk about all the dumb things people say about menopause that bother us. Our teams assist us as we maintain the balance needed to experience a meaningful and healthy life change. Menopause does not have to be a chamber of horrors. (NOTE: MAP/Calibration can, in like manner, be helpful for achieving and maintaining balance during the menstrual cycle, as well.)

Also, I have asked in MAP/Calibration sessions to receive understanding about what menopause really is for us and how to better understand and view it. For me, this has sidestepped the assumptions, myths and medical misknowledge that are associated with menopause. I must say that this experience has been deeply rewarding, and I recommend it to other women.

I also recommend this kind of MAP/Calibration to men who would like to understand more about what is really happening with their partners and how they (the men) fit into this picture.

A related point for men: Their chemistry also changes when they are in their forties and fifties. MAP can assist men with these changes, as well.

The following is an article written for our newsletter *Perelandra Voices* by a woman who worked with her team on the issue of estrogen replacement therapy.

*My gynecologist put me on estrogen therapy about two years ago. A competent physician, and respectful, he suggested I kinesiology test the regimen—the frequency, not the dosage.*

*I am unhappy taking manufactured hormones. So I asked my MAP team, "Do I need to take the hormone today?" and got a positive. Now I check every day. I record when the answer is negative and when it turns positive. The hormone has a palpable effect. I always feel better, but I just hate taking medicine. My team indicated I would be on this regimen for months. So I set up a log to keep track.*

*Prior to involving my MAP team, my physician proposed two weeks on and two weeks off. But I became grumpy and miserable on the two weeks off. Since I teach, I didn't want to take it out on my students. So I tried it two weeks on—one week off. No luck. After day three, I was miserable. Finally, the light dawned. I asked my team; and behold, I got help. My most sincere thanks to you, your associates and the Perelandra staff for making access to these new dimensions.*

J.R., Pennsylvania

The next article from the *Voices* newsletter is by a woman who worked with MAP for a gynecological problem.

*I have been greatly helped by MAP. I had been spotting at mid-cycle for a year. I wasn't concerned because it was minimal and occurred only at ovulation. Then one day I had heavy bleeding and cramping in my cervix. This did make me take notice. My body was trying to tell me something that I needed to address. I immediately opened a MAP coning and was told to test for flower essences and have a MAP session. I cannot describe how comforted I felt during this entire four- to five-day process. I was assured I didn't need medical treatment. I also understood this was a healing process to release old trauma from my body.*

*Fifteen years ago, I had been biopsied for cervical dysplasia. As I was in the MAP session, all the emotions held in at that time came to the surface. I sobbed with the pain of feeling so alone during that ordeal. I also relived the humiliation of the procedures. I was literally almost yanked off the table during the biopsy. The tissue did not want to be taken out and yet the doctor insisted on doing that. Then there were the follow-up treatments of tissue being frozen (cryosurgery) and later cauterized. I felt awful about being disconnected from a part of my body, angry at my partner for the lack of support, frightened and humiliated by the procedures. And I had a terrible sense of loneliness. As this overwhelming loneliness arose, I asked to be comforted so I would not feel so alone this time. I truly felt I was held in loving arms. I still had to feel the pain, but there was not the isolation that had previously existed. I was told to meet the next morning for a MAP session. This continued for four consecutive days. Each day we met for a MAP session, I received the healing support of my MAP team and the flower essences. By the end of the four days, the bleeding had subsided and the sensations of pressure and cramping in my cervix had pretty much abated.*

*There were lessons to learn as I saw the flower essences that came up. I saw areas of my life where I was asked to take more responsibility for myself. I could see connections that had to be made for healing to occur.*

*I felt very much at peace during this healing process. My attention was drawn inward, and I felt able to be with my body and not be fearful about what was occurring. There actually was a feeling of sweetness about it: the amazing support and love I was receiving, the sense of coming back to my body, and of being able to nurture this very traumatized part of myself. I often had spontaneous images of a very healthy cervix come up. The support I received allowed me to feel the absolute naturalness of this unfolding process so I was able to cooperate fully and easily.*

*This is the first cycle I have had since this experience. I am so pleased that I did not have any breakthrough bleeding, the first time in fifteen months! I can honestly say that I can feel a difference in this part of my body. The trauma has been released. My MAP team and I just celebrated the anniversary of our first year, and I feel honored and pleased to see myself entering more and more into a co-creative relationship with them. I appreciate the perceptual changes that allow me to take more responsibility for myself and contribute to healing the planet.*

M.L., California

I added the following editor's note with this article:

Make sure you feel comfortable and at ease about *not* seeking regular medical help when your MAP team says it's not necessary. This is only a suggestion from your team. If you would feel more comfortable going to a regular physician, do it. If nothing else, the visit will put your mind at ease.

Just prior to the doctor's appointment, open a MAP coning. Tell your team where you are going and the physician's specialty, if he or she has one. Ask the team to monitor your visit. Then, right after the appointment or sometime later that day, have a MAP session and let your team continue the physician's work in ways that are appropriate for you.

If you don't have a MAP session immediately after returning

from the doctor's office, ask your team if you should close down the MAP coning. They may wish to continue monitoring you, depending on your reaction to the visit and the state of your health. If they wish you to leave the coning open, find out how long it is to stay open. Then close the coning at the appropriate time.

If your team does not need the coning to be left open, close it down after you return home and re-open it later when you are ready to do the "post–doctor's" MAP session.

## Accidents and MAP

You've had an accident. You are still conscious, and you must go to the hospital emergency room. Take ETS Plus right away and open an emergency MAP session. The full process is given in Chapter 6 and the easy-reference steps are in Chapter 8. I recommend that you read Chapter 6 several times to become familiar with the process so that you can recall it in an emergency without having to dig for the book. You might even open the Emergency MAP coning several times just to practice. And make sure you have your ETS Plus easily available for emergencies.

While you recuperate from an accident, have frequent MAP sessions. If you can't get scheduling information from your team because you can't do kinesiology testing and/or can't hear them, just have a session each day as you move through the initial recuperation stages. Also, tell them what therapy you are getting because of the accident.

● EMERGENCY MAP FOR OTHERS IN NEED. The full process and information for setting up or surrogating a session for someone else who is in an emergency situation is in Chapter 6. It's easy to set the session up for someone, but there is one major, ethical issue: You must have the person's *conscious* permission to set up the session. You cannot throw a MAP team in someone else's lap. Nor can you throw someone unwittingly into MAP's lap.

If you feel you would like to offer MAP to someone in need, if the chance should arise, take time to think about how you would explain MAP to someone else who doesn't know about it or wouldn't normally be attracted to such a thing. Be careful about what words you use. Make it short, to the point and inoffensive. Try it out on others a few times and modify your explanation according to the reactions you get from these people.

● IF A PERSON IS IN A COMA. It is just as crucial that you receive permission from them as it would be if they were conscious. Here's what to do: Treat the person as if he/she was conscious and fully capable of hearing you. Explain MAP. Speak audibly and softly to the person. Then set up for surrogate kinesiology testing and ask simple yes/no questions. "Do you understand what I'm explaining?" "Would you like me to explain it again?" "Would you like me to set up a MAP coning for you?" If the answer to the last question is "no," you need to back off. If "yes," set up a surrogate Emergency MAP coning. (See Chapter 6 for the complete Emergency MAP steps.)

At one of the MAP workshops, a woman explained that her adult daughter had been in a coma for years due to a car accident. The mother began using MAP and felt that it was just the thing her daughter needed. She did not bother to explain

MAP or get permission from her daughter to open a coning for her. The best way to describe what happened when the mother opened the session is that the daughter fought it. She didn't know what was happening to her. So she became restless and agitated in extraordinary ways. The mother remembered what I had written about this situation and talked to her daughter about MAP just as if her daughter were conscious and could hear. Immediately the daughter calmed down. She's now out of the coma and talks to her mother about the things she sees her MAP team doing for her. And she can describe her team in detail, too.

The mother explained that she was talking about her experience in a public workshop because she wanted to make sure others, who have the best intentions, just as she did, pay attention to this permission business before opening a MAP coning for someone.

● Long–distance emergency MAP. Do not try to set up a long-distance surrogate Emergency MAP session for someone, even if you have permission. These sessions require that the person have support from you. You need to be in the room and ready to administer ETS Plus both during and after the session. To set up a long distance session basically leaves the other person in the dark and unsupported. It is not an appropriate thing to do.

● Setting up for emergency MAP. Many who work at Perelandra have also "joined" MAP. We have in their files the code name for their team in case there's an accident. In a family or group situation that is MAP-friendly, you might consider recording everyone's code name to use during emergencies.

## Keeping Your Team Informed

● TEAM UPDATES. Keep your team up to date on current health issues. For example, when a flu epidemic hits your area, tell your team. They do not keep themselves up on your current events. You will have to supply this information.

● THE THREAT OF A SERIOUS DISEASE. If you are frightened about some serious disease, or you know someone who has a serious disease or has died from the disease, talk to your team about it. (And talk to your friend who has the disease about MAP!) Even if you are not at risk, the fact that you have a fear about this disease can compromise your PEMS (physical, emotional, mental and spiritual) balance. And if you are in a situation where you are at risk, keep your team abreast of any feelings that you have. There is a strong link between your immune system and your state of mind.

Here is a personal example: Seven out of eight members of my immediate family died of cancer. Even though I have distanced myself from patterns that might have contributed to their cancer, and even though I have a good personal attitude and strength, I still hit an internal panic button if anything even slightly suspicious happens to me. I pay attention to those panic-button messages and I immediately inform my team. Just talking with them about it is helpful. But apart from this, telling my team about it is part of my responsibility to keep them well informed about what's happening to me physically *and* emotionally.

● EMOTIONALLY CHARGED QUESTIONS. I strongly advise that you not ask your team emotionally charged questions like, "Do I have cancer?" Your ability to accurately perceive their answer is questionable—whether you are using kinesiology or another method for "hearing" your team. In these situations, it would be better for you and your team if you got a sound diagnosis from a medical doctor whom you trust. And, just like the allopathic doctors tell us, MAP also feels second and third opinions are valuable. Your team already knows if you have a serious problem. It doesn't need the diagnosis. However, it needs your cooperation and understanding of the situation in order to effectively work with you. Getting a diagnosis that has been verified by one or two other doctors moves you through the process of receiving a good foundation of information from which you can work with your team. It's an invaluable education process for you and will help you ask the right questions and give the right information to your team as you move through a treatment program. Also—and this is equally important—it removes the doubts from your mind. You know what your diagnosis is, and you are not self-diagnosing or assuming a diagnosis based on what you think or hope your team is saying.

● IF SEASONAL FLU or any other contagious illness is flying through your family and you want to avoid it, tell your team what's happening. Nine times out of ten, they'll keep you from getting it. If it's unavoidable, your downtime will be shorter than it would be for those who don't use MAP.

● GETTING SICK. If you become sick, I suggest that you have a MAP session daily. Among other things, the team can move you through the illness quickly. Your downtime will be much shorter. However, your symptoms may be more intense than you would normally experience. This is happening because the team is making sure your body processes the illness efficiently. Continue doing MAP sessions along with any other health regimens you work with. Do what's needed to be comfortable—and blow your nose often. You'll be out of the illness faster than you could imagine possible.

## Consulting Other Health Care Professionals

I've written that you need to tell your team what therapists and physicians you are seeing. Then your team can work in conjunction with them. Also, it is good to open a MAP coning before you have your appointment. This way, your team can monitor what is being done for you. Take ETS Plus right after you leave the doctor's office. Then, as soon after the appointment as it is feasible, close the coning and take ETS Plus again. Be sure you talk about the appointment in your next session so that your team will know how you feel you were affected.

● CHIROPRACTORS. If you see a chiropractor when you need adjustments, for example, your team will assume that you *prefer* to have your chiropractor make them. The MAP team will not override your decision to include someone else in your overall health team.

Although a MAP team is perfectly capable of doing chiropractic adjustments, they will not automatically do so in this situation. They will either tell you to see your chiropractor or assume you will see him on your own. If, from time to time, you want MAP to do the adjustment, you must specifically request it. There is no competition going on here. Your team will respect your preferences.

● ENLARGING YOUR MEDICAL TEAM BEYOND MAP. If you have been diagnosed with a serious illness, don't limit the scope of your treatment by ignoring alternative and quality allopathic options and just focusing on MAP. Let your team assist you in choosing the best combination of options the medical community can offer you. If you are battling a serious illness, you want to attack the problem from every angle and every level. The MAP team concentrates its work in two areas: (1) it assists you and helps you coordinate the available options as you seek to put together the best possible treatment program, and (2) it works directly on your body, emotions, mind and soul in conjunction with the full treatment program and in ways that are unique to MAP. In short, by including MAP as a major part of your treatment program, you will ensure greater efficiency and effectiveness as you work to reclaim your health.

## Emotional Therapy and MAP

I think the best way to get across to you the value of working with a MAP team for emotional issues or while you are working with a therapist is to let people who have had this experience describe it.

*My therapist thinks I'm a whiz kid at psychotherapy. She can't understand how I so rapidly moved through my therapy and so quickly brought needed changes into my life and began using them. Little did she know that I did a MAP session before each therapy session and fairly often another MAP session afterwards. I'm sure with MAP plus flower essences I got through it in one-third the normal time.*

*In therapy I have come to see how I survived my childhood by parenting my parents. I learned to disengage the active, powerful, intelligent parts of myself so that I could maximize the supportive, nonthreatening, nonquestioning side of my nature and be the dependent child they needed. Even though I've progressed quickly with this issue, when I'm with my parents the same "dismembering" of myself still occurs if I'm not watching carefully—right before my eyes.*

*During a recent visit, at the time of my son's graduation, when I needed to be functioning well, this began to happen. I escaped to the bathroom and opened a MAP session. I explained exactly how I was feeling; I said I was feeling very afraid because I had incapacitated myself to protect my parents, but that this left me feeling helpless and insecure and, of course, angry. I was afraid that my insecurity would lead me to hurt them and spoil the occasion.*

*Lying on the floor of the bathroom, under a towel, a change occurred. When I emerged, I was again in contact with myself—strong, together, fully functioning, no longer angry and able to enjoy the rest of the visit. The hectic day went by very smoothly and was actually enjoyable for everyone. To me this was a major miracle.*

M.B., Maryland

*Being in a new relationship has brought up old issues for me around boundaries, violation, fear of abandonment, etc. MAP and I have moved entire patterns out of my body and psyche by stating my intent to let the pattern go and follow directions. I connected with the White Brotherhood "incest recovery unit"* and in half an hour moved out a pattern that* *had plagued me for years. The energy of violation left, as did three men who were inappropriately connected to my energy system. For several days, I felt like my "clothes" were too big for me. There was so much space in my body. And, when making love, it was my energy only in my body for the first time.*

*I've also had a big destructive "fear of abandonment" pattern come up in response to my partner's healthy need for more time and space to himself and less frequent sexual encounters—finding the balance. So we did a coning and I was told I was using sex as the antidote to fear of abandonment and what I really needed was to anchor the pattern of unconditional love. So, one by one, I went through every relationship where I'd felt rejected and abandoned, forgave that person, asked for forgiveness and experienced unconditional love. It took several days of essences to stabilize this work. I have a whole new outlook on how my partner and I use our time together and apart, and it is wonderful!*

M.L., Ohio

*For doing specialized work such as incest recovery, simply connect with your MAP team in the usual way, inform them what special situation you would like to work on, and request that you have the appropriate members on your team for this work. This may be a modification of your personal MAP team, and you need not have a separate code name or symbol for them. Just connect with them within a regular MAP session by making the above request.

*I had returned from an out-of-state funeral for a friend of mine. He was a young man with a wife and four small kids. He died in a totally unexpected and tragic way. It was a full military funeral. My being around the grieving relatives and friends, and the ceremony affected me deeply. I had been sad about it before, but when I got home it was as if I had picked up the grief of everybody and brought it all home. It felt as if it were impregnating my uniform and clothes. I felt a hollowness inside. I felt emotionally stunned. I couldn't concentrate and get on with my life. So I had a MAP session and asked for help in getting past that. As soon as the session was over, I felt totally cleared. I still felt sad at losing my friend, but I was free of that smothering cloud of grief and my life was back on track. This felt like a miracle.*

E.R., Oregon

## MAP Options: ETS Plus, Flower Essences and Kinesiology

● ETS PLUS AND FLOWER ESSENCES. When I wrote about MAP in the first and second editions, it was important that people understand the value of using flower essences in conjunction with the program. At MAP workshops, before ETS Plus was developed, I asked people who began the program without using the essences and then included them later, if the essences made a difference. Only once did someone say no. Everyone else talked about how much clearer the sessions were for them once they incorporated the essences. They also talked about how much more efficiently and quickly they were able to feel the results of the sessions. And many said their ability to hear and sense their team improved tremendously.

Now we have ETS Plus. It is easier to use than flower essences and requires no testing. Consequently, ETS Plus has replaced flower essences as an option in the steps of MAP sessions, and it provides you with the same results. This gives those who didn't want to learn about flower essences and how to test them the chance to get support for their MAP work by taking ETS Plus. And it gives everyone else who has diligently tested flower essences as part of their MAP sessions a wonderful break. No more testing!

But flower essences are still important for MAP people, as seen in the above comments. Just because we are now recommending ETS Plus for MAP sessions, I wouldn't want anyone to shy away from considering adding flower essences to their health regimen simply because they think essence testing is complicated or hard to learn. It is neither. Essences provide important and sometimes necessary support over a long period and valuable feedback for the root issues we are dealing with.

In Appendix C, I describe ETS Plus and flower essences. If you wish to learn about flower essences and how to test them, I recommend the video *The Human Electrical System and Flower Essences* and the book *Flower Essences.*

• FLOWER ESSENCE CHEATING. Some people have tried to get around the issue of learning to use flower essences properly by emptying all the essence bottles in their sets into one jug, and taking a swig of this at regular intervals. Ahhhh—nice try. They need to take ETS Plus instead. Creating an essence cocktail only complicates matters. By taking all the essences at once, you require your body to cast off the ones that aren't needed. This is what the body does naturally with essences that aren't needed. You are now putting an additional burden on yourself. Plus, by taking a sip from the all-purpose jug, you don't know which essences you actually need, and you don't have any input as to how you are reacting and responding both to the work and to the specific issues that are being worked on. You have eliminated a useful feedback tool.

• ETS PLUS VS. FLOWER ESSENCES. To clarify, you test for flower essences after you close the coning and have taken your three doses of ETS Plus. If you then test that you need essences, this means that you would benefit from additional support for the MAP work over a longer period of time.

● KINESIOLOGY. You do not need to know how to do kinesiology to do MAP. However, as you develop your relationship with your team and the work, you will most likely want to ask specific questions about different issues. Kinesiology gives you the ability to bridge to your team. You ask them a simple question in a yes/no format. They project the energy of a "yes" or "no" into your electrical system. You do the kinesiology test on your electrical system, and from this you discern if the team's answer was "yes" or "no."

As I mentioned earlier, if you are overwhelmed at the idea of learning kinesiology or you are having problems with it, bring it up to your team and ask them to help you over the hurdles. You'll be surprised how fast you can learn to test!

I have provided updated steps for learning kinesiology in Appendix B. If you run into any problems learning the technique and you are having trouble catching the help your MAP team is providing you, just call our Question Hot Line. We'll be happy to get you over the hurdle.

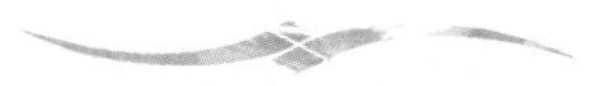

## Helpful MAP Aids

● KEEPING NOTES. Take notes on the sessions. Record the difficulties and problems you talked about, sensations you felt during the session, and results you perceived after the session. At some point down the road, these notes often reveal patterns we had no idea existed. They also help confirm to *ourselves* that something really is happening in MAP, that it's not our imagination. And sometimes we go into a period of MAP work when we feel nothing during the sessions. We swear nothing is happening. We even entertain the notion that perhaps our team has walked out on us! But it's just that the work they are doing is, for the time being, on levels we can't perceive physically. Everyone in MAP experiences this at some point. When it happens, just continue with your session schedule. At some point, the team work will shift and you will once again feel things during the sessions. In the meantime, a casual review of the notes reminds us that, indeed, these sessions are for real.

● PERELANDRA SUPPORT. We offer a video of an extensive MAP workshop I gave at Perelandra. It's cleverly titled, *MAP —The Workshop,* and it includes eight hours of information. Many people purchase this video set and hold MAP evenings with friends who also wish to learn MAP. This not only gives them the information they need to get into the program and to use it well, but they end up with an automatic support group of friends, as well. The workshop covered material for new people to MAP as well as fine-tuning material for people who have been using the program. (See p. 203.)

We also have a Question Hot Line that you can call for information and answers to any questions you might have. And you are welcome to email questions to us any time.

See the contact information in the back of the book for getting more information on the video and the Question Hot Line.

● GROUP SUPPORT. When *MAP* was first published, folks told us that they wished they had someone to share their experiences with, but no one near them had ever heard of MAP—or wanted to hear of MAP. Now there are many people using MAP, and it's not so hard to put together a support group.

We offer a special networking list for MAP people. If you wish to be on the list, email us or drop us a note and let us know. This makes your name and address available to others who are in your area and want to talk with someone about MAP. If you would like a list of people in your area who are on the networking list, email us or send us a note about this, too. (You don't automatically get information about others in your area just by requesting to be put on the networking list.) We will send you the list.

The following is a *Voices* article about one MAP support group. We titled the article "MAP Anonymous."

*As a practicing registered nurse, I see a huge potential in MAP. Ultimately we are all responsible for our own health. MAP gives everyone easy and simple tools to do just that. Western medicine does not yet have a true understanding of who does most of the work concerning health and wellness. It truly is not the doctor or nurse, acupuncturist, herbologist, chiropractor, or massage therapist, etc. It is each of us individually. MAP provides us with the necessary knowledge. To work directly with MAP is quite a profound honor. Thank you for starting me on such a wonderful journey.*

*In January 1992, I received a surprise letter from another flower essence user in my area. She requested we get together for sharing and learning about MAP and flower essences. I had taught her childbirth several years before and had no idea she knew about flower essences. On February 9, 1992, we had our first gathering . . . four women. We came with a wide range of life experiences, diverse educational backgrounds and lifestyles. It was wonderful. We talked for hours. I would like to share some of the common experiences we had while using MAP.*

*1. Since January and February of this year, a lot of us noticed strong sensations of pressure or pain/tenderness in the head area, frequently at meridian points or along the natural suture lines of the skull. Each of us was surprised at having similar symptoms at the same time!*

*2. During the early sessions, some of us saw an extraordinary green color, not previously seen. It was an almost fluorescent hue.*

*3. Each of us had been given what we felt was confirmation of our connection with nature during the early sessions. Our experiences were different and totally unexpected. As an example, immediately after my first session with MAP, as I opened my eyes, I saw brilliant, beautiful, green letters on the ceiling. I distinctly remember reading them one by one, as random letters. It wasn't until nearly an hour later that I realized the letters were P-A-N. The realization was quite profound.*

*4. Each of us had an awareness of MAP workers coming into our energy fields and leaving. Some members initially experienced the exit of the team as quite abrupt and jarring, but not painful. When we requested that this be less abrupt and smoother, in the next session for each of us it was!*

*5. Each of us had a feeling at times of cold/shivering during the sessions.*

*6. Each of us had a pattern of essence use with MAP: lots of essences needed after a session, but next time a few. This was an alternating pattern.*

*7. Most of the group received verbal (audible) or intuitive help via conversations during MAP.*

*8. Some of us just experienced the physical presence of our MAP teams through sensations in our bodies.*

*9. All of us experienced complete relaxation and a feeling of wholeness during a session, and a desire not to end that session, or to have another session soon to experience that place again!*

*10. All of us have had nothing but positive, pleasant healing experiences using MAP.*

*Our small group tries to meet monthly to share experiences and gain reinforcement and encouragement regarding MAP.*

*We all seek the full understanding of who we are and how we can maintain, improve, or regain optimum health by using ourselves, and reaching into that all-powerful inner source.*

*Our families often ask about MAP. Some have been very receptive and are using the process. Others quietly observe and accept our choices without wanting to participate in any way. . .yet!*

*In all this, we are each learning our own inner truths, and gaining support and companionship from our group and our MAP teams. It helps to maintain a good sense of humor when we challenge ourselves with family strife, job uncertainty, parenting issues, or health problems. This support is reinforced for all of us at each gathering.*

J.H., Massachusetts

## A Note of Caution about Sharing MAP with Others

Many people who have success with MAP suggest the program to their friends. Please—be sure that when you make the suggestion, you are prepared to share your copy of *MAP* with them. Or buy them their own copy to give them when you make the suggestion, if you don't want to let go of yours. Do not, under any circumstances, just give them the easy reference steps in Chapter 8. Worse yet, don't just tell them the steps. Everyone who gets into MAP needs to be fully informed. And they need the information to be unfiltered. This is so they can develop their own relationship with their team in a balanced and safe MAP environment.

NOTE: MAP may be the best thing to have ever come along for you. Your life may have changed in dramatic and exciting ways since you started the work. Because of this, you may have a burning desire to share MAP with everyone you know—and maybe even some you don't know. I ask you to be sensitive when sharing MAP. If you don't know for sure that the other person would be comfortable with this information, be caring and considerate about sharing the information with them.

## What Does Not Happen in a MAP Session

Some of these things I have already written. But I think they bear repeating.

You are in control of the coning at all times. The MAP teams do not open a coning on their own. *You* must do this. And the teams will not refuse to close down a coning. Once you indicate a coning is to be closed, it is closed. The teams will not ignore or override your requests. Also, your coning is protected. Nothing more needs to be done to "shore it up." However, someone who has paranoid tendencies or extreme victimization problems should not enter into the MAP program. They will not be able to accurately discern what is happening to them and will automatically turn MAP into a frightening experience. If such a thing is happening to you, stop using MAP immediately, and work on your personal issues in ways that don't set up an automatic fear response. No matter what, MAP cannot protect you from yourself.

MAP is a medical program. It is also a *human* medical program. MAP is not intended for animal care. (See Chapter 11 for the *Nature Healing Coning for Animals.*)

The MAP teams are not hoodlums. They do not kill your begonias or steal your money. Although you will experience love and respect from your team, they will not say things like you are the only one who can save the world—then proceed to give you a long list of wacky things to do for saving said world. These are all self-conjured experiences that spring out of fear or a deep desire to "live a significant life." If you are having such experiences or are "hearing voices" that say strange things and won't stop, tell your team and let them help you regain your balance.

## AN IMPORTANT MESSAGE FOR ALL MAP USERS

Over the years we have become aware of several people who are running around telling others that there is a "new MAP," and they just happen to be the one chosen to inform everyone about the MAP changes. They've even said that the MAP teams haven't yet told me about the changes. Then they proceed to scare the bejesus out of people by telling them things like they are being attacked and taken over by aliens and the MAP teams want them to keep their coning open twenty-four hours a day for the rest of their lives. Here are some facts about MAP that I hope will put you at ease.

● The head of the MAP program is Lorpuris, the head of the White Brotherhood Medical Unit. I speak with him daily. He's not going to change the MAP program without telling me about it. It's not as if we don't talk to one another and he hasn't gotten around to telling me this news.

● Map has a built-in protection. It was decided prior to the program "going public" that any changes or modifications would come through Perelandra. This is not because we at Perelandra claim a monopoly on MAP. It is to avoid confusion among MAP users. Without this coordination anyone could announce changes to the program, and everyone would have to figure out whose changes were legitimate and whose were not, creating a fair amount of chaos in the program.

● Map was designed to accommodate the wide range of approaches that are needed for the many different people who participate in the program. In part, this was done so that the teams would not have to modify the program for a long time. MAP has not become obsolete and the teams do not anticipate needing to change it for many years to come—certainly not in our lifetime or in our children's lifetime . . . or in their children's lifetime.

● INDIVIDUALIZED CARE. Because MAP is set up to meet individual needs, it is not unusual for one team's approach and work to be quite different from how the other teams work. It is important that we not confuse what is unique about our personal MAP work and think it is what everyone else needs to do or that it is a sign of wholesale changes in the program.

● VICTIMS OF MAP SCAMS. If you know someone who has been "taken in" by would-be MAP changes, suggest to them to go back to using the program as it is outlined in the book. They need to talk to their team about the frustrations they are having with MAP that made them open to suggestions to changing the program in the first place. When someone deliberately attempts to shift the MAP session setup outside the structure of the program, their team will not continue to work with them. Instead, whenever a MAP coning is opened the team will attempt to bring the person back to understanding what MAP is about and stabilize the person until he is ready to participate in the program as it has been set up. No matter how hard a person tries, he cannot manipulate a MAP team to operate in ways the team does not wish to operate.

If you have gotten caught up with someone else's ideas about how MAP should be used and you are still confused after reading this, please email or call us at Perelandra right away so that we can help you get back on track.

## ENCOURAGEMENT FROM OTHERS

In 1989, I introduced MAP during a workshop. The folks were given the steps and encouraged to try the program. Several months later, I sent out a letter asking them for feedback as to whether they were working with MAP and what their experiences were. Out of fifty workshop participants, thirty responded that they were now working with MAP. They gave me permission to use portions of their letters so that others could benefit from their experiences and thoughts. There are a lot of references to flower essences. This was because ETS Plus was not yet available.

Several of the letters are from our newsletter. I'm including these because I feel they also say something that will both assist and support you.

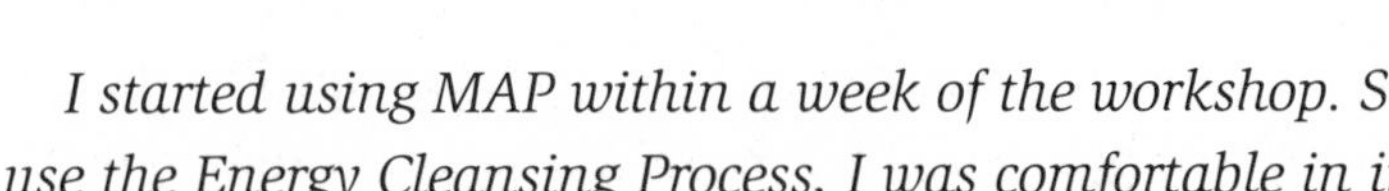

*I started using MAP within a week of the workshop. Since I use the Energy Cleansing Process, I was comfortable in invoking the four participants in the MAP coning. I'm not a little awed and humbled at the generosity of the Deva of Healing, Pan, the WB Medical Team and even my Higher Self, in making themselves so readily available.*

*I find it easy to talk with them and joke with them. For example, while I picture that they are working on me to help me physically accommodate spiritual expansion, I tell them that helping me relieve myself of some cellulite around my thighs would also be very welcome. I tell them about emotional issues I'm working on (e.g., resentment, aches and pains I've got, chronic tight sore throat, aching joints, how my eyesight is changing rapidly), what events are going on in my life (e.g., my kids both have a bad case of chicken pox, my spouse is living across the continent with no plans for returning). I feel energy moving in my body during the sessions, particularly at the base of the spine and up my spinal cord. I also feel sensations in my neck, head, shoulders, pelvis and the bottoms of my feet. It seems to me so far that the more I give them immediate feedback as to what I'm feeling, the faster the next sensations come. It's been pretty amazing, but never overwhelming. Frequently, I am relieved of aches and pains I had when I first lay down.*

*The biggest "problem" I have is finding the privacy and time for the sessions. (I'm essentially a single parent of an infant and a kindergartner, and I work and I'm forty-one years old. Age gives me an edge on wisdom perhaps, but physically the child-rearing is harder.) I have even gotten a babysitter to have sessions.*

*What I feel overall from the sessions is that they are fine-tuning me physically and energetically, and I have an increased general sense of well-being. I feel emotionally nurtured from the sessions. And it seems they work very well with the other healing and spiritual work I am doing.*

*I have had a few sessions unlike the others. During the first two of the unusual sessions, I fell asleep—it was irresistible and I felt that it was okay with my MAP team. I was jolted awake (a big, soft jolt) with a flash of white light in my chest. I pictured the team with the energy equivalent of one of those heart machines that are used to shock people's hearts into restarting. It was a surprising sensation, but not unpleasant.*

*The third session I want to tell you about felt like a non-event by contrast, at least initially. I wasn't aware of any sensations, energy moving, etc., as usual. I considered that I was not having a MAP session. As I lay there though, I realized that what I was labeling as "mental drifting" was much more vivid and meaningful than that. It felt like I was getting a lesson from my unconscious or right brain, and the pictures were in fact helping me to understand the issue I had asked my team to address at the beginning of the session.*

B.G., Florida

*I was not ready to do this kind of work for a long time. I respected that as an indication that the timing wasn't right for me yet. I also think I wasn't yet ready to make the commitment to go through whatever changes would be involved. However, during the past holidays, I began to feel that the time was right to begin.*

*My scanning session seemed fairly uneventful. I had the sense nothing was happening yet, other than everybody getting acquainted. I did get my symbol when I asked. An image of a torch popped into my head as soon as I asked.*

*I have been doing the sessions twice weekly, but have just gone to a once-weekly schedule. My normal time to do them is about 8:00 P.M. I start by making the coning connection as you outlined. I keep a notebook handy and record the essences and any issues and experiences that come out of the session. I do the sessions in bed, usually with a pillow under my legs. . . . I set a timer in the kitchen for forty-five minutes, and then go into the bedroom. By the time I connect, test for essences and get into bed, about forty minutes are left for the session. Usually, I sense that the session is winding down a few minutes before the timer goes off. I thank everybody, close the coning and retest for essences.*

*I have felt very little physically while in the sessions, including the initial scanning session. There has been no pain or unpleasantness so far, except for one session where I felt very restless and found it hard to be still.*

*I think the main issue we've been working on has been an emotional one, centered around my self-worth. Often, I start the session drifting off into sleep, only to awaken suddenly with some image or flash of insight, and a sense of clarity and light about who I am and what I'm doing here in this present life. It seems like maybe the drifting off is the way we have of getting my day-to-day mind out of the picture for a while so that the rest of my mind can say something to me. I do feel that the insights are coming from me, and that MAP is facilitating the process.*

*I have had a couple of more physical experiences. Once, I felt embraced by a very warm and loving being, in an aura of total acceptance. It was an immediate kind of thing, not something airy-fairy. Another time, I felt like I was filled by a clear, bright light that made me buoyant. Both of these only lasted for seconds, but were so strong that the feelings lingered way past the session, and actually return whenever I remember them.*

*It took me a couple of sessions to get used to doing it, but now I make a point of verbalizing what issues I'm bringing into the sessions and what I'm experiencing during it. . . . Speaking makes things clearer to everyone involved.*

*The main word I have for how the MAP team works with me is "unobtrusive." I know they're there and I feel things happening, but it's subtle. It's like they take their cues from me and never force anything. The image I have is that exercise where two people face each other and one makes movements that the other duplicates, so that the first person feels like he's looking at his image in a mirror. It's that sensitive quality I feel from the team.*

*After almost two months of sessions, I have to say that MAP is very helpful and really pretty easy to do, once you make the commitment to do it. I have felt more clarity in my life and a greater sense of being connected with a larger reality. I credit MAP for some of the moves I'm making in my Feldenkrais work. I've found that MAP doesn't eliminate any issues or any work on my part but makes it all flow better. I have this image of the team squirting all the creaky, rusty joints of my being with oil to make them work smoothly.*

C.W., Virginia

*Yes, I have been using MAP; and, yes, it is a test of faith. I needed to address lingering issues of self-worth first—i.e., the belief that my life and work are not "important" enough in the universal scheme of things to "deserve" such specialized medical treatment. I knew from the moment they began surfacing that these thoughts were/are erroneous, but the more deeply anchored feelings accompanying them kept me from contacting MAP and requesting their services. Working through these feelings eventually led me to realize the significance of the law of free will and also Jesus' statement "Ask and you shall receive."*

K.W., Michigan

*My basic issue centers around feeling comfortable with something that is beyond my five senses. I have experienced subtle body sensations, seen energy patterns swirling in front of my eyes, and gotten hunches that I should do things, but I still sometimes get angry at myself that I don't experience these sessions with greater conscious awareness.*

*Interestingly, in spite of not feeling competent about my ability to sense what's going on, the initial scanning session seemed very real to me. I needed essences to start the session. I got my team's name easily. . . . I saw something that I interpreted as my team's symbol (a swirling circle of energy that was also pulsating and contained a number of brilliant points of light or stars). I also felt some tingling in my arms and legs as if energy were being run through them.*

C.P., Virginia

---

*After I attended your workshop, I knew immediately that I had to work with MAP. The problem that I have hasn't been helped in twelve years with medical practice. The scanning session went well. I felt energy going up my spine and head area. At times I felt back pain, neck pain and was uncomfortable. I received no symbol.*

*During my first session, I spaced out several times. They were spinning my head around (a very strange experience!), working on the cranium. Also they spun my hands around and worked on the hands. Then I was given a symbol.*

*Oddly enough, in the beginning I bought a little notebook and recorded everything in it. Alas, it came in handy.*

*I have no fear about this work, but then I perceive mostly through intuition. Sometimes I feel like an idiot lying there for forty minutes talking to the air. At that point I'll say, "Please give me a sign you are there. I feel so dumb." And then I would feel someone brushing against my forehead or hair. Without doubt, I know that someone is there with me.*

R.S., Pennsylvania

*Scanning session: I was very excited and curious to start the process. . . . I felt a little awkward not knowing who or what I was talking to. I felt the presence of four—three males and one female. I asked if that was correct and received an affirmative. For most of the first session I just listened and "felt" what was happening. I did feel a lot of movement, pressure, all around me, especially around my head and abdomen. I would occasionally describe what I was feeling and ask if it was them. I would always receive an affirmative reply by kinesiology testing.*

*For the rest of the sessions, meaning up until now, I haven't perceived the presence of anyone but continue to feel the energy sensations—although at times it is so subtle that I sometimes wonder if it is all my imagination. Close to the end of the first month, I started asking for some kind of confirmation. That is when I started "dreaming" a lot.*

*The only consistent part of the sessions has been that no matter how hard I try, or the time of day or night of the sessions, I always fall asleep if for only the last few minutes. Then I will wake up only to find the session over.*

*Regarding how I have felt changes: I "feel" that I am in some kind of "process" that I can't really articulate, but I feel comfortable and good about it. I feel a seriousness about the process—don't know if it's me reflecting back to me or if I am actually perceiving the team to be a really serious team. A little kidding around would be welcome—I think.*

J.B., Virginia

*MAP arrived "just in time." When I ordered it, I had no idea that I would need it. Yesterday I wondered when I would start the program. Today, I knew, and it was now.*

*Soon after entering into the session I became aware of an almost weightless sensation and remember thinking "This is amazing. I expected to be one of those people who wouldn't feel anything and would have to go on faith." Then I had a strange sense of being turned, but not completely over. Soon after that, I was aware of an energy taking over my right hand and working with it. I figured this had to do with the trauma and consequent condition of my hand ever since my wrist was broken in 1985.*

*The next area my team worked on was my left hand. A month and a half ago, I told my chiropractor that I feared I was getting arthritis in my hand, and she examined it and said that a small bone was out of place. She corrected it and it improved at once. I hardly ever noticed anything with it anymore. My team worked on it for quite a while—longer than on any of the other areas.*

*At some point not too far into the session, I suddenly wondered what my symbol would be. Immediately "White Lightnin'" came to mind. That seemed inappropriate. "That can't be it," I thought. "I think that's one of the Rose Essences."*

*The areas I would have chosen for my team to work on, they did not choose. At least, to my knowledge they didn't. The second half of the session seemed uneventful, though I remained awake and alert. When the hour was up and I asked for my symbol, "White Lightnin'" came and nothing else. I was still doubtful, but said "Okay."*

*When I was writing the report of the session in my journal, it occurred to me to look up White Lightnin's definition. I was amazed and thankful, too. Suddenly, this symbol seemed perfect.*

H.H., Pennsylvania

*I'm a physician's assistant. A few months ago I reread your book* Behaving... *and then got on your mailing list. When I read about MAP, I knew I had to do it. I found* MAP *in a nearby bookstore, and this process has transformed my life more than I can describe. I want to tell you of some of my MAP experiences.*

*I was so excited when I found the* MAP *book that I read it in one sitting and wanted to do everything immediately. It was the answer to my prayer in many ways. The next day I did the scanning session. I told them I was willing to give everything to this, I was ready to break out of my limitations, transform my life, and move as fast as I could while still being able to cope with my outside life. Man, they took my word for it! The scanning session was incredibly intense. After a few minutes, I felt I was being sedated, as if I were getting pre-operative medications given patients to make them groggy. I felt whooshes and rushes of energy in various places, and gentle probing and dissection, almost. I had very intense pain in one hip joint that gradually increased in intensity. I felt as if my bones were being remodeled. I didn't have problems with that hip before—just weird muscle spasms as a teenager. It was an exhausting and amazing experience. After the hour, I was drained and somewhat shaken —but had no doubts that this stuff was real! The pain in my hip continued for one more hour and then was suddenly gone. I thought, holy cow, if this was the scanning session, I don't know if I will live through a therapeutic session! But for the next several days (I did it daily), the sessions were very gentle.*

*My sessions go through phases—lately I feel nothing at all, but there is a periodic humdinger. Sometimes I "blip out" through some or most of the session. At times I feel the most extraordinary sensations. Either energy or parts of my body are being scanned in grid works, as if they are being peeled off layer by layer, or just being touched. Sometimes I see things in my mind's eye, energy moving from place to place or funneling like tornadoes, or clear images of objects or places. Sometimes I feel the compassion, love, support and enthusiasm of my team. This has made such a difference in my life. One of the greatest benefits to me is feeling I do have a team—a group of beings I can talk to and work with who care about me and help me. It eliminates a lot of the loneliness in life. I have studied and practiced many spiritual disciplines. But so many of them have such a gap between the inner experience and the outer life. With my MAP team, there is such a concrete, easy and practical way to integrate everything in my life with my life purpose, deepest desires and philosophy. Before this, I had felt so frustrated, stuck and discouraged. I had hit a wall and didn't know how to get any further. Enter the MAP team! I don't have to know how. I just needed to be willing to change and do my best. And things have been changing, so easily and almost unnoticeably. From little things, like night-time foot cramps that I haven't had since I began the program, to seeing myself relating to people much more openly and freely, to my life once more being filled with happy coincidences and small miracles. I have seen changes happen on every level that I had assumed would take years of agonizing work.*

*Everything in my life isn't healed. I still have stuff to deal with, and new stuff comes up all the time. But now there is a way to actually work through it and not wallow in it for the next twenty years. Another change I see in my life is that I used to get sick when things began to be "too much." I'd get sick and it would give me an enforced reprieve and rest. Now when I start to feel myself getting sick, I can see why I'm doing it. Also, I choose to work with why I'm feeling overwhelmed instead of just taking a breather. And I'm not getting sick anymore. When I began the MAP sessions, my initial emphasis was on physical stuff, but very quickly the emphasis switched to basic issues like life purpose and my relation to the world.*

E.R., Oregon

The following is from a physician who is using MAP.

*This whole method of healing works on the electric/energy body level, I think, which then impacts on the physical over the next twenty-four hours. I can't think of a single thing it has to do with the allopathic medicine in which I was trained. However, I am a member of the American Holistic Medical Association, a group of physicians who are connected by their common desire to find a truer form of healing than the concept of the mechanistic (Newtonian) body, which we were taught in medical school. I think there are people in that organization who would be interested in this, and I am asking for guidance from my team on the proper place, time and person for presenting this to that group.*

*I'm impressed that MAP is so easy—when I meditate it takes great effort and concentration to move my mind to "another place." With MAP I make the request, focus rather lightly on the coning and the team, and things just happen. Since it is a process that takes care of itself so easily, I think the most helpful thing for people to overcome fear and skepticism would be to read about others' experiences. I do know in my practice I have had to learn that some people do not want to be healed; similarly, MAP won't fit into everybody's needs or present state of growth. The beauty of it is, when one is ready, all one must do is ask for it. Truly a case of ask and you shall receive.*

A.R., Arkansas

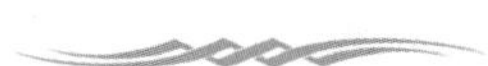

*Chapter 5*

# *The MAP/Calibration Process*

EARLY ON IN MY WORK, NATURE came up with a brilliant process that is designed to balance us when we are having difficulty moving through times of emotional and mental stress. I began working with this process immediately and found that the Calibration Process can be easily combined with MAP sessions. Although the Calibration Process is an excellent tool to be used on its own, I have found that the MAP/Calibration combination is even more effective.

First, let me introduce the Calibration Process to you as it was given to me in a nature session. Included are my comments about working with the process. Then I'll explain why it can and should be added to MAP and how you can do that.

## SOME PERSONAL COMMENTS ON THE CALIBRATION PROCESS

I worked with this process extensively for nine months after I translated the Calibration Process session in March 1990. I wanted to understand and experience it before offering it to others, and I wanted to explore the different ways in which the process could be used. From the very first time I worked with it, I was amazed. I would like to pass along to you some of my feelings about the process and give you ideas about when it can be used.

What impressed me first was the efficiency of the Calibration Process. It only takes a half-hour once you've explained the problem. Initially, I questioned this, not believing that so little time was needed to accomplish so much. In all of my work with the Calibration Process, the sessions have not exceeded the time it takes to express the problem and the half-hour. I'm quite used to nature coming up with exceptional co-creative processes that redefine the concepts of efficiency and effectiveness, but I was still impressed.

It took a little thinking on my part to figure out when I was in a situation that could be helped by the Calibration Process. It is *not* needed if we are moving through an emotional or mental process where we have a sense of forward motion being maintained. It's useful when we feel our wheels spinning or feel stuck and can't even begin to imagine how to proceed—in other words, when we're at a dead end. The Calibration Process does not sidestep emotional and mental processes. It is designed to keep our processes moving on all of our levels and "unjam" those places where we seem to have gotten stuck.

The first time I used the process was in March 1990, when I knew I was having difficulty addressing my work in the garden and maintaining focus on what I needed to do. I had tried every trick I knew that might "wake me up." I felt my ability to focus return, but it was short-lived, and I would quickly sink into what felt like a hole. I decided to try the Calibration Process. I set it up exactly as it was written in the session. I tried to explain as simply and succinctly as possible how I was feeling and how my life was being affected. And I admitted that I knew nothing else I could try. I sat for the half-hour and felt nothing happening. I closed the coning as instructed, assuming something would occur that would tip me off that I was now "healed" or whatever. Since I had done this session in the evening, I went about my "off hours" as usual. I still noticed nothing different by the time I went to bed. The next day, I began my day without thinking about either the process or possible changes. I just got on with what I had wanted to do. By the end of the day, it occurred to me that not only had I accomplished everything I could have hoped to do and more, but I had done all of this effortlessly. Not once did I feel I had to deliberately press myself through a project. I simply did it.

I wanted to share this first experience with you because it shows so clearly how the process can work without a bunch of bells and bugles sounding. In this instance, one day I was in one state of being (a difficult, unconstructive, wheel-spinning state) and the next day, after doing the process, I was in a completely different state of being. I didn't experience a linear progression from the first state to the next. I simply found myself there. Sometimes I have found in this process that there aren't any great and glorious moments of understanding and resolution. At times I have felt that the gears between my emotional and mental levels and my body are simply "off" and in need of a little calibration. So, nature gets everything back into sync, and the blocks that seem to cause the wheel-spinning unjam, and that's all it takes.

At other times, I did go through a resolution and understanding process that occurred either within the half-hour or within the twenty-four hours after the process. Again, it wasn't like some baseball bat hitting me in the head. Nothing that dramatic. I'd be moving along in my day and suddenly I'd know what the troublesome issue really was. Usually that in itself was the resolution. Or sometimes the resolution was in the form of action I needed to take to resolve the issue.

I have used the Calibration Process when I was mentally buzzing and couldn't stop, when I couldn't stop working, and when I could see that a fear I was experiencing was actually counterproductive and not helpful. Or, for some crazy reason, I found myself unable to make a decision even when I had all the information and input I needed.

Another example: When I give a workshop, I work with the Calibration Process in two ways. First, a week prior to the workshop, I ask to be calibrated for "workshop preparation" for the specific class. This puts me in a receptive, reflective, creative state, and helps me prepare the workshop in new and better ways. Second, twenty-four hours prior to giving the class, I have another calibration for what I call "workshop go." This calibration shifts me out of the more internal, reflective preparation state to the external presentation state. Their dynamics are very different, and I find that by using the Calibration Process, I am able to shift into each state with greater ease.

Everything I have experienced from this process verifies to me what nature says about the need to strike an involution/evolution balance within ourselves in order to function well—that is, working with nature and myself as a team. All my calibration experiences have been accurate, efficient and effective. In working with the process, I have grown and developed in the area of emotional/mental balance in ways that allow me to see more clearly new areas where this process could be useful.

One of the first things I suggest to others as they learn about the process is to have a series of calibrations around the issue of understanding what constitutes emotional and mental situations that could benefit from calibration. I find that most of us limit our definition of emotional to pain we experience in relationships and don't understand mental issues at all. I had to expand my own understanding before I realized that I could calibrate something like learning difficulties or persistent physical problems that have an overlay of mental and emotional issues I'm not aware of. Now if I suspect a Calibration Process would be helpful, I'll open the coning that is used for this process, and ask: "Is this a situation that could be helped with the Calibration Process?" So far, I've always been told yes.

The following is the session from nature that introduced the Calibration Process to me those many years ago. It includes the steps for working with the process independent of MAP.

## UNDERSTANDING THE ISSUES HUMANS FACE AND WHY IT IS IMPERATIVE TO CREATE CONSCIOUS PARTNERSHIPS WITH NATURE

*It is becoming increasingly important for humans to understand the extensive partnership they have with nature, especially when focusing on issues of form and consciousness and all that this combination implies. We are in an interesting time in human development where the desires and needs of the human soul on Earth completely outstrip the ability of the present support frameworks. By this we mean support frameworks in all areas: agriculture, science, physical health, mental and emotional health, government, social, education. . . . The development of the human soul collectively on Earth has surpassed the development of its support systems. In the nature-dominant environment that existed on the planet prior to 1932, the human soul could more easily develop support systems that were compatible. One reason for this is that nature was abundant and could accommodate every human's needs. (We do not mean to imply that all needs were met, only that all needs could have been met had humans so chosen. The physical means for all human support could have been met at any time because of natural abundance.)*

*Since then, this balance has shifted and the planet has become human-dominant. Nature is no longer abundant enough to accommodate human needs and desires without careful consideration regarding the larger picture. We don't see this as a "bad" development. If ignored, however, it would be a dangerous development for all. But it is also a development that is forcing the human soul to expand on every level in order to address and survive the severe challenges that the shift to a human-dominant planet has created. Prior to this shift, individual human souls could expand and develop in ways that were not associated with survival. In short, there was a sense of leisure around this kind of expansion. The individual had a lifetime to expand his understanding from a broader perspective, while at the same time he devoted his efforts and energy primarily to those activities that served to support his day-to-day physical survival. Now, for the sake of survival on all levels, the human soul is required to make this shift, this expansion, and to do it quickly.*

*The present support systems were designed to best address human survival in a nature-dominant era that existed within a Piscean context (parent/child emphasis). Now the shift to a human-dominant era is being affected by the Aquarian impulses (partnership, balance and teamwork emphasis). All of the previously workable support systems are crumbling. At the same time, humans are expanding. By this we mean that the human in the conscious state is expanding to enfold the human spirit in the unconscious state. With this fusion, when it occurs, the unconscious becomes conscious. Humans are beginning to understand in an immediate and personal way that life is far broader and more complex than they ever before understood. This expansion does not occur in a vacuum. It requires support on all* PEMS *levels (physical, emotional, mental and spiritual) in order for it to be stabilized and maintained. So humans are expanding in their efforts to address serious survival issues on all levels, while at the same time they are having to function within a collection of frameworks that were never designed to meet the pressures of the present issues. There is an ever-expanding gap between today's expanding human and the planet's various social support systems' capabilities.*

*We have not gone off the topic of presenting the co-creative Calibration Process. We are giving you the background needed to understand the crux of the issues that humans face as well as why it is now so imperative for them to link in conscious partnership with nature in order to develop the support systems of the future—and we mean the near future!*

*The expansion of the human system requires that the expertise of nature in the areas of the relationship of five-senses form to energy and involution (bringing spirit and purpose into form) be tapped in direct proportion to the expansion. In your vernacular, the intensity and complexity of the game have increased to such a degree that the relative simplicity of the old support systems has been rendered ineffective. Humans must become partners with nature in order to establish the systems that will support the new complexity. Don't forget—the expansion of human consciousness to enfold its own unconsciousness includes the grounding of the entire expansion into form. Otherwise, the expansion will either falter or take on an ungrounded air and be useless. This expansion process is what is referred to as "the evolution dynamic." The grounding of the expansion and its expression through form is what is meant by "the involution dynamic." The human soul is being pressed to open beyond or soar above the existing support systems on the planet in order to see the new. To properly support this expansion, the development of systems enfolding the balance between the involution dynamic and the evolution dynamic is imperative.*

*And this is what nature can give you now. It understands the relationship of energy to five-senses form, and it knows what is required in order for the direction and purpose of spirit and soul to become perfectly seated into form in balance. As we have pointed out a number of times, nature is the master of involution and the expert in matters involving the relationship of energy to five-senses form. In order to create support systems that respond to this new demand of human souls seeking to ground a broader picture of reality into form, man must turn to nature.*

*We do not mean to imply that if man turns to nature for the needed development of his support systems that this development will be effortless or perfect. We have no intention of perpetuating a parent/child dynamic in our relationship with mankind. We have no intention of dictating structure and process. In fact, this would be impossible. Humans must supply intent, purpose, direction and need when it comes to systems development. With this definition, we in nature will seek to supply the best structure in which to ac-*

*commodate and move intent, purpose, direction and need. It is a true partnership we seek. We will not interfere with or attempt to alter the human evolutionary thrust. We are here to assist and accommodate this thrust.*

*In medicine, humans have seen the relationship of nature to themselves in the areas of nutrition, natural medicines and stress relief. Humans do not see themselves as nature/human soul systems requiring involution/evolution balance. Instead, they see themselves as souls utilizing nature for the purpose of evolutionary growth. Nature has been the servant of the soul while the primary thrust of the human has been evolutionary. This cannot and does not work. The human system itself is a partnership between soul and nature, and its thrust, its primary focus, is the involution/evolution balance. When in form, and we mean by this any existence within the band of form, the human must strive for involution/evolution balance in order to achieve evolutionary movement. Without this balance, there is no evolutionary movement, activation, or change. The involution dynamic is the tool of the movement, activation and changes required by the evolution dynamic.*

## THE ARENA OF EMOTIONAL/MENTAL HEALTH

*First, let us say that we refer to this arena as "emotional/mental" because the dynamics causing a person to be classified in need of emotional or mental assistance are, from nature's perspective, the same. The distinction between the two is created by humans and does not concern nature.*

*You will recall, Machaelle, from your personal exploration in this area that when you came upon an emotional block that seemed impossible for you to get through, you asked nature for help. We will say now that the insight to ask for help was, in fact, initiated from us (nature) and in response to our desire to assist you in any way possible. You picked up on this insight and acted on it by opening a coning with the intent for us to assist you. It is essential that people understand that in areas where nature links with the human, it (nature) can only do so on request. We do not assume a partnership. To do so would be to override human free will and thus render the human powerless. This would be against universal law, and nature, on its own, does not live or function outside universal law.*

*As you told us what your emotional situation was, we observed the energy dynamics as they shifted and moved throughout your system on all* PEMS *levels. (We see the human system on all* PEMS *levels because that complete system is functioning in a form state.) We were able to observe the emotional blocks you were struggling with from the perspective of energy. From these observations, we were able to alter the blocks as well as the general movement of energy in a way that assisted and made more efficient that energy's movement. In short, we assisted you in achieving involution/evolution balance in those areas where you had temporarily lost it. As a result, you experienced the shifts, insights, releases and understanding required in the reestablishing of involution/evolution balance throughout your entire system. Remember, we see these blocks from the standpoint of energy—what is moving appropriately and what is not. We see your system as consciousness relating to form from the perspective of involution/evolution balance. We do not define what results in insight, understanding and resolution. This is the evolutionary input for which you are responsible.*

*Our process with you is an example both of the partnership we seek with humans and how we can work together in every way to achieve full, inspirited, functioning form. Where the will of the human is present, and where we of nature have been requested to help, we will adjust, shift and facilitate the involution systems in order to support the human's evolution process. For us, it is a relatively simple matter to work with you in this way. In fact, it is solely a matter of receiving a person's request for our assistance.*

*We suggest that we work together using the following process.*

[NOTE: Where essences are used in the steps, ETS Plus may be used as an alternative. In fact, ETS Plus is required if you are not using essences. Take one dose of ETS Plus instead of testing the essences.]

## THE CALIBRATION PROCESS STEPS

1 *Open a Healing Coning: Overlighting Deva of Healing, Pan, a link with the White Brotherhood (state that you would like the appropriate link with the White Brotherhood for a Calibration Process), and your higher self.*

*NOTE: We recommend that flower essences be used in this process. We suggest that the person first test for essences after opening the coning and prior to stating the problem. This will stabilize the person throughout the process. A dosage need not be tested for, since any essences needed in the beginning of the process will be for short-term stabilization.* [Or, take one dose of ETS Plus.]

2 *Request assistance with a problem on the emotional or mental level, or a problem on these two levels that is connected and physically manifested.*

3 *State the problem. State it as if you were telling a therapist. Talk about the problem itself and how it is affecting you physically, emotionally, mentally and/or spiritually.*

4 *Once you have given a full description, allow yourself a half-hour to move through the stages of insight, release, understanding and resolution.*

*NOTE: You may not perceive any changes in attitude or understanding during the half-hour. This will be because the process of shifting understanding and changes in attitude sometimes needs to move through more complex levels in order to reach a point where one can perceive the effects. We suggest that if you sit quietly for a half-hour and no sense of understanding or resolution has come to you, simply move forward in faith that within twenty-four hours you will experience understanding, change and resolution.*

5 *We suggest that you test for flower essences again just prior to closing the coning and include a dosage/solution test for continued support during the post-calibration integration period.* [Or, take one dose of ETS Plus. Then, if you wish, test flower essences and dosage for any needed additional support.]

6 *Close the coning by stating you would like to be disconnected from each member of the coning, one at a time.*

- *Your higher self*
- *White Brotherhood connection for this Calibration*
- *Pan*
- *Overlighting Deva of Healing*

*Test, using kinesiology, to make sure the coning is closed. (If you test negative after asking if it is closed, refocus on the coning and again request to be disconnected from each member, one at a time.*

*You simply lost your focus the first time. After the second time, you will test positive.)*

● *ADDITIONAL NOTES. We see some emotional/mental problems as comparatively complex layers of energy movement. It is quite possible that for the* final *resolution of an emotional/mental issue, one will need to go through this process several times—that is, a calibration* series. *As you move through the series, you will receive one insight after another. Each will serve as a building block for the foundation that is needed for the final overall resolution. But we stress that timing is a key factor. If and when a follow-up session is needed, you will sense something related to the original problem that has become an issue. One need not plan ahead for these follow-ups, for you will need time between sessions to integrate the insight, release, understanding and resolution from the previous session. As you move through this for each session, one layer of the problem will be eliminated or resolved and the next layer will surface, and new questions or issues will come up. Have another calibration session as the new questions/issues are raised.*

*In these more complex situations, you will be moving through a series of sessions with us that will resemble the Peeling Process or Two-Week Process described in the book* Flower Essences. *As we have said, you will move through one layer at a time, experiencing a sense of resolution after each layer, which, once integrated, will signal you to move on to the next layer.*

*The half-hour timing covers the time span we need to move the human system through involution/evolution imbalance into involution/evolution balance.*

*For twenty-four hours after a calibration, you may feel tired and a little quiet—you may even feel an ache or pain that has seemingly popped up from nowhere. These are simply reactions to the calibration and should be gone within twenty-four hours.* [Taking ETS Plus and/or] *the flower essences solution from the post-calibration integration-period will assist and stabilize you greatly through this twenty-four-hour period. However, if a reaction should persist, set up another Calibration Process around the same issue and explain all of the various reactions you are having. Nature will do additional adjustments that will either move you through or eliminate the reactions.*

*The Calibration Process is an additional nature-partnership procedure that is not in and of itself strictly a flower essence process. With or without the essences, this process can work. Flower essences* [and ETS Plus] *would be most helpful, however, in stabilizing you throughout the Calibration Process itself and afterwards during the time needed for integrating the work accomplished during the process.*

## THE MAP/CALIBRATION PROCESS: COMBINING CALIBRATION WITH MAP

In regular MAP sessions, the White Brotherhood Medical Team is working directly with you, and they take the primary lead in the session. Nature is supporting you, assisting your team and stabilizing the team's work. When used in MAP, the Calibration Process is used at times when the healing process is best served by nature taking the lead and having the White Brotherhood medical team in a secondary role to support and assist nature's work.

There may be times when you wish to combine the Calibration Process with MAP. The steps in this third edition for a combined MAP/Calibration session are different from what I wrote in the second edition of MAP. This is the updated information that is now recommended when working with MAP. This additional information is also in the Perelandra Video 4: *MAP—The Workshop.*

● SETTING UP. You can initiate a Calibration Process within a MAP session or your MAP team may suggest you set one up after the session has begun. If you know you're stuck on something, you can go into a MAP session and immediately tell your team you feel stuck and that you would like to set up for MAP/Calibration. Or, you may already be in a regular MAP session when you realize that the issue you are addressing may require a Calibration. Or, you're in a MAP session and all of a sudden you hear your team say or you get the idea that they want you to do a MAP/Calibration.

> Ask, *Do you want me to do a MAP/Calibration?*
> Test, using kinesiology.
> If you get a "yes," set up for a MAP/Calibration by saying, *I'd like to set up for a MAP/Calibration, and I'd like Pan to shift forward.*

Your MAP team will immediately shift, and the White Brotherhood members will go into a secondary position while Pan takes the primary position for the thirty-minute Calibration Process.

● YOU ARE NOW IN THE CALIBRATION, and you just start talking about the mental and emotional elements of the issue you were discussing or having a problem with. Follow the directions for explaining the problem that are outlined earlier in this chapter.

● YOU TALK FOR THIRTY MINUTES. Or, if you don't have much to say, you talk for ten minutes and leave the Calibration open for the remaining twenty minutes. In MAP/Calibration, the process takes thirty minutes *total,* and that's all it takes.

● ENDING THE CALIBRATION. At the end of the thirty minutes, come out of the Calibration by saying,

*I'd like to close the Calibration, and I'd like to shift Pan back to the MAP focus.*

Now the White Brotherhood team shifts forward and nature moves to the secondary position, in the support role. Wait five seconds for the shift to occur and then take another dose of ETS Plus.

● MAP/CALIBRATION SESSION TIME. With MAP/Calibration, you are required to devote *seventy minutes* to the full process. The MAP session is forty minutes, and the Calibration takes another thirty minutes.

- If you were ten minutes into your MAP session when you started the Calibration Process, when you come out of the Calibration you now have thirty more minutes to go in your regular MAP session.
- Or, if you were fifteen minutes into a MAP session when you switched to the Calibration, you spend thirty minutes in the Calibration and are then required to spend twenty-five minutes in the regular MAP session to complete the process.
- The MAP session can be split into two segments, but the Calibration time cannot be split.

● MAP/CALIBRATION "EQUIPMENT". You or your team can call for a Calibration anytime in the MAP session, so be sure you have a clock, ETS Plus, pen and paper with you when you start a MAP session. If a Calibration is needed, note the time you spent in MAP before the Calibration, so you can figure how much time you need to continue the MAP session following the Calibration.

● ETS PLUS. To work with the Calibration Process, combined with MAP or on its own, you will need to use ETS Plus to stabilize the work. For this process, ETS Plus is not optional.

● THE ADVANTAGE OF MAP/CALIBRATION. Again, in Calibration, nature is doing the work, and your team is observing and supporting. There is an advantage to doing the Calibration in MAP and to having MAP session time after the Calibration. When you give your team this additional time, any follow-up that is required as a result of nature's work can be done by your team.

● UPDATE ALERT! In the second edition of *MAP,* I recommended that you automatically set up the Calibration Process within all your MAP sessions. With the new refinement in the session process presented in this third edition, I no longer recommend that. Sometimes it is best to do just a regular MAP session and sometimes a combined MAP/Calibration is called for. But remember: When you do add the Calibration Process, the teams now prefer this new setup (thirty-minute Calibration plus forty-minute MAP session). This keeps the process more precise and provides additional support to you.

If you are not sure when to add the Calibration Process and when to do a regular MAP session, just tell your team the issue you wish to address, ask about Calibration and test to find out if it is needed, using kinesiology.

## THE MAP/CALIBRATION STEPS: UPDATED

1 OPEN THE MAP SESSION as usual, activating the MAP coning.

- Overlighting Deva of Healing
- Pan
- Your White Brotherhood Medical Team
- Your higher self

2 SETTING UP THE CALIBRATION. When you wish to switch to the Calibration Process, tell your MAP team that you are making the switch and state:

*I'd like to set up for a MAP/Calibration, and I'd like to shift Pan forward.*

Wait five to ten seconds for this switch to complete. Pan, who is already a part of the MAP coning, will automatically shift from that coning dynamic and move into a connection with you that is appropriate for the Calibration Process.

3 TALK ABOUT THE DIFFICULTY you are experiencing and feeling stuck on. Say everything that comes to mind about this issue. Allow thirty minutes for the full Calibration Process.

4 SHIFTING BACK TO MAP. At the end of the thirty minutes, close the Calibration Process and shift back to the regular MAP coning. State:

*I'd like to close the Calibration, and I'd like to shift Pan back to the MAP focus.*

Wait five seconds. Take one dose of ETS Plus.

5 COMPLETING THE MAP SESSION. Continue by completing your regular MAP session.

6 CLOSE THE CONING. When the MAP session is complete, close down the coning as usual. Disconnect from:

- Your higher self
- Your White Brotherhood Medical Team
- Pan
- Overlighting Deva of Healing

Wait ten to fifteen seconds.

7 TAKE ETS PLUS TO STABILIZE THE SESSION. For this, you will need to take *three doses* of ETS Plus. Take the first dose immediately after closing down the coning. Wait five minutes, then take the second dose. Wait five more minutes and take the final dose. This will stabilize both the MAP work and the Calibration. Spend a few minutes quietly before going on with your day. NOTE: In MAP/Calibration, you take ETS Plus *after* the coning is closed. In a regular Calibration Process, you take ETS Plus just before closing the coning.

- STUBBORN AND CHRONIC ILLNESS. As explained, the Calibration Process can be used anytime you feel stuck on an emotional/mental issue, feel like you are going in circles, not getting anywhere and you are spinning your wheels. Here's something else to consider: If you have a chronic illness, it's a safe bet there is an emotional/mental aspect to it that must be processed for full recovery. The illness may be chronic because there is a problem with how you are processing the mental/emotional elements, and nature needs to calibrate something. For chronic ailments, ask your team if you need to do MAP/Calibration around this issue.

## ENCOURAGEMENT FROM OTHERS

*I have always been interested in psychic phenomenon and have never experienced such, except dowsing. It is, therefore, with some incredulity that I experience the results after using the MAP/Calibration Process. Not only do the things that seem to be getting in my way get resolved, but often there is an accompanying insight. An incredible tool!! Thanks a thousand times!*

R.L., California

*I began using MAP/Calibration and the flower essences about six weeks ago. My attitude to the processes can best be described by that old Biblical statement "Lord, I believe—help thou my disbelief." My mind was open but my faith marginal. Over the past weeks, my belief is gaining ascendancy over disbelief.*

*I presented the MAP/Calibration team with a chronic (twelve years or so) neck stiffness, a source of ongoing discomfort and frequent headaches. I had previously sought relief by a host of modalities including chiropractic, yoga, relaxation and visualization exercises—and resorted mostly to aspirin.*

*After two weeks of MAP/Calibration and flower essences, the neck stiffness was much improved. Now it is gone.*

A.G., Pennsylvania

Here's a suggestion for using the Calibration Process on its own from an article written for *Voices.*

## The Group Calibration Process: *Updated*

by Clarence Wright

*The Greek philosopher Heraclitus once said, "You can't step into the same stream twice." That wise philosopher used the stream as a metaphor for ever-changing life. Forms and structures never stay the same. Things occur; stuff happens. Just when we think we know the rules of the game, the whistle blows and the rules change. If Heraclitus were alive today, he'd probably be struck by how fast today's streams move.*

*Even though change is necessary for the evolvement of new and better forms, it sure can throw us for a loop. Today, rapid change occurs in businesses and other organizations where people work together for a common purpose. To be effective, organizations need to enfold new energies and constantly recreate themselves. What we're talking about is a change of form to more effectively meet the organization's new needs.*

*I'd like to share with you the Group Calibration Process we use at Perelandra to deal with changes in our form in two areas: integrating new employees into the organization and helping all of us work more in sync with each other and with Perelandra's overall purpose. Like other organizations, we are undergoing much growth and change. While this is exhilarating, it can at times stress us out and leave us scratching our heads and wondering what we are doing. The Group Calibration Process has been invaluable in creating an atmosphere of mutual support so that everyone can contribute fully to the work being done. It has been a great help in keeping us focused on why we do what we do, as what we do changes. It also makes available to us the assistance of nature, the acknowledged expert in form change.*

*The Calibration Process is a way of directly involving nature in change and making it maximally effective. It oils the gears and adjusts the screws to keep us from jamming up when undergoing change. What I would like to explain is how we use the process in a group setting and what it has meant to us. Any group whose members desire to work in a co-creative manner should find it helpful.*

*One person acts as facilitator for the group and leads everyone through the following steps of the Group Calibration Process.*

1 *All individuals in the group take one dose of ETS Plus (ten to twelve drops) for general balancing before starting the group calibration.*

2 *The facilitator opens a Group Calibration Process coning. The points of this coning are*

- *the Deva of the organization or group,*
- *Pan,*
- *the appropriate connection with White Brotherhood for a Group Calibration Process, and*
- *the higher self of each individual doing the calibration.*

*After the coning is opened, each person takes another dose of ETS Plus. Since the coning creates a new, temporary energy field around all those present, it's possible that a person may need help adjusting to that new energy.*

3 *The facilitator states the purpose of the calibration, such as bringing a new member into the group or the group's expansion into a new area of work, or the group's need to work more cohesively as a team.*

4 *The floor is opened to anyone with thoughts or suggestions about what related areas the calibration should address. It's important that everyone be clear about the purpose of the session. It is also important that each group calibration cover just one issue. If more than one issue needs to be addressed, plan for a series of calibrations.*

5 *Everyone then sits quietly for about twenty minutes, or until the facilitator tests that the session is complete. The facilitator can tell when people feel it is over by noticing increased fidgeting and moving around. At the end of the quiet period, the floor is then opened again for people's impressions, thoughts, images, etc. This is where we have gotten some of our most useful information about what current changes will mean for our group. Sometimes people come up with similar images.*

6 *At this point everyone takes another dose of ETS Plus to help in grounding the information that came up during the calibration.*

7 *Finally, the facilitator closes the coning, expressing thanks to each of the elements that made up the coning. Once again, each person should take a final dose of ETS Plus now that the energy of the coning is gone.*

8 *There is an eighth step that I highly recommend. Finish the meeting with some great chocolate cake or a fabulous lunch, topped off with espresso or a pot of tea. For us, this inspires some great sharing about the calibration in a very relaxed atmosphere. Be sure to have someone keep notes on the main points that come up.*

*The Group Calibration Process works so well because it focuses everyone's attention on the issue at hand. With nature's help in the process, people notice how grounded and solid the information is that comes out of the session. After all, nature is the master of grounding. And the best thing is that nature doesn't charge a red cent for the service! It's free for the asking. (Be sure to make your financial officer aware of this last point!) Also, nature makes house calls at any time, twenty-four hours a day.*

## A HEADS-UP FOR PERELANDRA ESSENCE USERS

With the release of the book *The Perelandra Essences* in June of 2011, the Calibration Process was upgraded and streamlined for those who use the Perelandra Essences. The new process is the "Basic Telegraph Test for Mental and Emotional Issues." Instructions are given on pages 214–215 of *The Perelandra Essences.*

Approaching mental and emotional issues this new way provides a broader, more comprehensive and stronger treatment regimen. You'll come out of it with a deeper and longer sense of stability on all your PEMS levels. If you use the Perelandra Essences, I recommend using these updated steps.

*Chapter 6*

# *Emergency MAP Procedure*

USE THIS PROCEDURE FOR severe trauma caused by accidental injury, sudden severe illness, or sudden emotional trauma. I suggest that you practice opening this coning and "working" the process several times until you are comfortable and confident that you can do this in an emergency. Just be sure to let your team know you are going to do a few practice drills. It's best to memorize the steps, since you will not want to be rummaging around looking for them in the book when you're in an emergency situation.

You will be working with your personal MAP team. Obviously, then, to use the Emergency MAP Procedure, it will facilitate the process to already be in the MAP program, have a team and a team identification code.

## OPENING EMERGENCY MAP: UPDATED STEPS

1 Simply state: *I want to open an Emergency MAP coning with the __________ team.* (Insert your team's code.)

It is important to open the Emergency MAP coning *and* connect with your personal MAP team. The coning includes nature's stabilization, and the code name immediately links you to your MAP team. No special focusing is needed to open an emergency MAP session. Just make the above request (aloud or silently), and it will automatically happen. There is no need to wait ten seconds after this connection. This is a special setup designed to be used in serious situations when you can't afford the time it takes to open a regular MAP coning, and you can't focus on anything but your emergency situation anyway.

Once you are connected with the coning and your team (which occurs immediately), proceed as follows:

2 If available, take one dose of ETS Plus (ten to twelve drops) every three to five minutes for the first twenty minutes.

3 Continue taking ETS Plus every thirty to forty minutes for the next two to three hours and get to a hospital as soon as possible. If you do not have ETS Plus on hand, don't worry about it and just get yourself to a hospital. Your team has been working to stabilize you from the moment you opened the coning.

4 Stay connected to the Emergency MAP coning and team during the trip to the hospital, in the emergency room and for however long you are hospitalized. The Emergency MAP coning will support both your needs and the hospital treatment throughout this entire period. You need not do anything special to ensure that this is being done.

- If you are hospitalized overnight or for an extended period, take ETS Plus four times a day throughout your stay.

5 Once you return home and before you close the Emergency MAP coning, ask your team how often you should do follow-up MAP sessions for the illness or injury. This may be daily, weekly, every two weeks—whatever is needed to move you through a complete recuperation. If you are too exhausted or weak to open a regular MAP session according to the schedule your team advised, request that the Emergency MAP coning remain open for a few more days. By then, you should have the energy to open and close the regular MAP sessions, and you can close the Emergency MAP coning. State:

*I'd like to close the Emergency MAP Coning.*

Optional: Once you close the Emergency MAP coning, take *one dose* of ETS Plus.

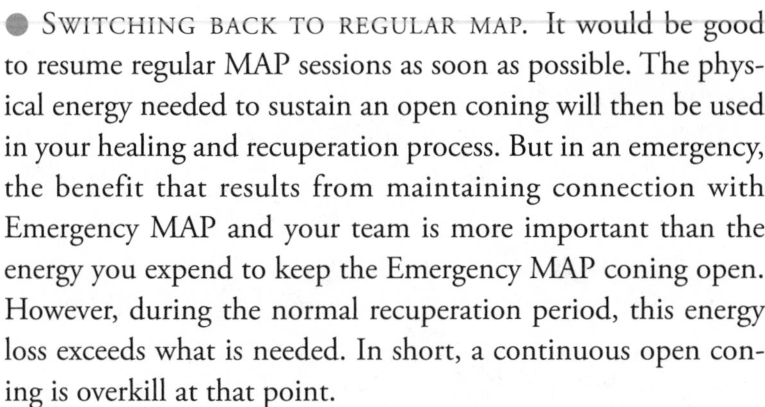

● SWITCHING BACK TO REGULAR MAP. It would be good to resume regular MAP sessions as soon as possible. The physical energy needed to sustain an open coning will then be used in your healing and recuperation process. But in an emergency, the benefit that results from maintaining connection with Emergency MAP and your team is more important than the energy you expend to keep the Emergency MAP coning open. However, during the normal recuperation period, this energy loss exceeds what is needed. In short, a continuous open coning is overkill at that point.

● KEEP YOUR EMERGENCY MAP TEAM INFORMED. While the Emergency MAP coning is open, you may talk to your team at any time. If you react to medication or treatment, or become uncomfortable for any other reason, tell your team *and* the hospital staff how you feel. If you don't have privacy, you do not need to speak out loud to communicate with your team. However, it may be easier for you to keep focused on what you say if you whisper. During an emergency, you have two medical teams working with you: the hospital team and the MAP team. Keep feeding information to both of them. If you are explaining something to your hospital team, your MAP team will automatically "hear" it. You do not have to repeat it to them. However, if you are suddenly hit with severe pain or discomfort, tell your MAP team while you are waiting for help from your hospital team. MAP will begin to work on you immediately before the other team arrives.

## SURROGATING AN EMERGENCY MAP TEAM: UPDATED STEPS

Just because you know MAP is effective and the Emergency MAP Procedure is especially effective does not mean that you should run around opening an Emergency MAP coning for everyone in need. Each person has his own patterns in life. The MAP teams respect this and are careful not to impose MAP on anyone who has not given his conscious consent. The least we can do is demonstrate the same respect for others' free will, timing and patterns. So, please be careful when surrogating an Emergency MAP team for someone.

- Be physically present. It is important that you be with the person you are surrogating. *Do not attempt to surrogate an Emergency MAP Procedure long distance.*

## Opening Emergency MAP for Someone Who Already Has a MAP Team

1 If you know someone who already has a MAP team and needs an Emergency MAP coning opened but is unable to do it, you may do it for him. Just say the name of the person, and state:

> *I request that an Emergency MAP coning be opened and that __________ (person) be connected to his/her team.* (State or visualize the person's team code.)

● You don't know the person's team code. If the person is unable to give you his MAP team's code, request that a MAP coning be opened and that __________ (name of person) be connected to his team. This will take a little longer (about two minutes at the most) as opposed to an immediate response if the code name is used. The MAP team prefers that the code name be used so that no time—even two minutes—be lost.

## Opening Emergency MAP for Someone Who Does Not Have a MAP Team

If you know someone who is in trouble but does not have a MAP team, *you must obtain his permission to open an Emergency MAP coning.* If he is conscious, simply explain MAP and offer to help him in this way.

● Explaining MAP to others. I suggest that you spend a little time before an emergency occurs thinking about how you might explain MAP and the Emergency MAP Procedure to someone without making them die of laughter. It takes some thought, but it can be done. Make it simple and to the point. After all, in an emergency you don't have time to get into a deep philosophical discussion about the fine points of MAP. It can be as simple as saying:

> *I would like to link you with a White Brotherhood Medical Team, a group of knowledgeable souls that will assist in stabilizing you. The link is immediate and can help you through this trauma. You need do nothing except give me permission to assist the hookup.*

Just by saying "White Brotherhood Medical Team" it will give the person enough information to consciously decide if he wishes you to proceed.

● DON'T TRY TO SNEAK THE PERSON INTO MAP. If this kind of concept upsets the person, you don't want to get into the position of assuming what's best for him and overriding his life patterns by trying to "sneak" him into MAP. You cannot sneak a person into MAP. The teams will catch you every time. They can read the intent of the person you'd like them to work on. Without an okay, the teams simply will not do anything, and they will wait for you to close the coning. If the person in the emergency says no, you need to back off. As I've said, it is his option to choose.

● DON'T PREJUDGE SOMEONE. If you would like to assist in connecting him with Emergency MAP, just give the person clear, straight-to-the-point information so that he can make a decision based on his own gut reaction.

## The Person Is Unconscious

If he is not conscious, you still need to obtain permission.

● MAKE PHYSICAL CONTACT with the person. For example, you can rest his hand on your arm or leg. Ask to be connected to his higher self. Do this by simply asking!

*I'd like to be connected to _________'s higher self.*

Wait five seconds. Test using kinesiology to verify you are connected.

● QUICKLY EXPLAIN MAP and the Emergency MAP Procedure just as you would for a conscious person.

● TEST FOR THE ANSWER. In a simple yes/no format, ask:

*Is it appropriate for me to open an Emergency MAP coning for you?*

Test using kinesiology. This will work because you are now connected electrically with the person, and although he can't speak to you, he can still hear you and respond to what you are saying. You'll read his response electrically through the use of kinesiology.

● TEST RESPONSES. If you get a negative response, respect his wishes and disconnect from his higher self. *(I'd like to be disconnected from _________'s higher self.)* Then get him to a hospital.

If you get a positive response, state:

*I request that an Emergency MAP coning be opened for* _________ (person's name).

MAP will take care of the rest.

● Once they are connected, you need to release your physical connection with the person and ask to be disconnected from his higher self. State:

*I'd like to be disconnected from __________'s higher self.*

2 If available, administer ten to twelve drops of ETS Plus every three to five minutes for the first twenty minutes.

3 After the initial twenty minutes, continue administering ETS Plus every thirty to forty minutes for the next two to three hours.

• If the person is hospitalized overnight or for an extended period, it would be beneficial for him to take ETS Plus four times a day throughout his stay. If he can do this for himself, just leave a bottle with him.

● Being in a hospital, especially in an emergency room, will make it challenging (at best) to administer ETS Plus. The above steps are a guideline for during this period. How much you can do for yourself (if you are the one in trouble) or if you are the one assisting another will greatly facilitate the body's dealing effectively with the emergency. The MAP team will be testing and administering flower essences, but like the regular MAP sessions, there is often a twenty-four-hour "lag time" between when the team administers the essences and when they fully impact the physical body. Taking ETS Plus as outlined will stabilize the body during this critical time. Obviously, in an emergency fast action is essential. This is why taking ETS Plus yourself or giving it to an injured or ill person is strongly recommended.

4 Once the person is home or out of the emergency situation, *you* close the coning for him. *Don't forget to do this.* You must be with the person when closing this coning. State:

*I request that __________'s Emergency MAP coning now be closed.*

Optional: Administer *one dose* of ETS Plus.

At that point, if the person is interested in pursuing MAP, teach him how to do regular MAP sessions. (Giving him a copy of *MAP* would be helpful.) He will not have to do the scanning session since this was already done in the Emergency MAP coning. He will need to request a code name, however, to facilitate his personal MAP sessions.

## ETS PLUS, EMERGENCY MAP AND MAP

You may assist the integration of your team's work and shorten the period between the session and when the work fully seats in your body by taking ETS Plus as prescribed for each session. This is especially important during emergencies and when we experience trauma. Should you experience discomfort or fear during a session, take a dose of ETS Plus at that point as well. If you are already using essences during MAP, the essences and ETS Plus are interchangeable. However, using ETS Plus instead of essences will eliminate the need for testing during your sessions and immediately after closing the coning. When using ETS Plus in conjunction with MAP, testing essences after each session is optional. However, if you choose to test essences for additional long-term support, do so within ten hours of the MAP session. (See Appendix C, our web site and catalog for more information on ETS Plus and flower essences.)

## USING MAP FOR SCHEDULED SURGERY OR DOCTORS' APPOINTMENTS

You could say that the Emergency MAP Procedure is used for *unscheduled* surgery and doctor visits. However, MAP can assist scheduled surgery and treatment in your doctor's office, as well. For this, you don't need an Emergency MAP coning. Open a *regular* MAP coning prior to surgery or your doctor's appointment, tell the team what you are going to do and any concerns or fears you have. Allow the coning to remain open throughout the procedure. If the surgery requires hospitalization, keep the *regular MAP coning* open for the entire time and work with your team as outlined in the Emergency MAP Procedure. Close the coning once you have stabilized and have the energy to open regular forty-minute MAP sessions that will go on throughout your recuperation. After returning home from doctor's appointments, ask if your team wants to schedule follow-up sessions, then close the coning and take three doses of ETS Plus. (See Regular MAP step 4, p. 172.)

By including the MAP team during scheduled surgery or appointments, the team can observe what is being done, how you are reacting, and assist and stabilize you whenever needed. Also, if you include your team in these scheduled "events," you don't have to try to explain to them in a regular session what went on. They've already observed what went on. You only need to tell them how you feel about what went on.

HINT: MAP and ETS Plus are *really helpful* during scary dental appointments!

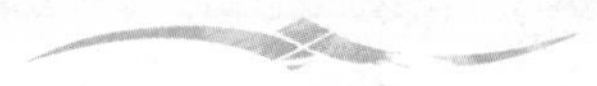

## ENCOURAGEMENT FROM OTHERS

ETS Plus is a new development, so you will read a lot about these people using essences with MAP and not ETS Plus. But just reading about the results people got from using essences will give you a good idea of the results you'll get should you choose to add ETS Plus to your MAP sessions. And reading about how they tested flower essences outside MAP for additional support for the MAP work will give you an idea of how to weave flower essences with MAP in the healing process.

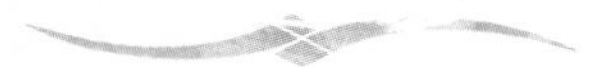

*In early April of 1992, I had an accident involving a sauna stove which I fell against from a pretty good height. My meeting with the stove resulted in first and second degree burns, a pretty deep cut and abrasion on the left side of my back, and a good amount of pain and shock. My partner had the presence of mind to locate a ride to the emergency room. She also grabbed the kit of Perelandra essences on the way out the door. On the way to the hospital, I opened a MAP coning and asked for some special assistance, and my partner tested me for essences.*

*After opening the coning and taking the flower essences, I immediately felt better. I was able to stay conscious and focused during our trip to the hospital and during the question-and-answer session in the emergency room.*

*While we were waiting for the on-call doctor to show up, my partner continued to test me for essences. She did separate tests for the burn, the cut and abrasion and the pain.*

*She and our friend who drove us to the hospital remarked at how fast the burn seemed to be healing. The blisters were actually shrinking before their eyes and the color of the skin around the cut was changing quite rapidly as well.*

*By the time the doctor showed up, an hour and a half later, the whole wound looked much better. The doctor cleansed and bandaged it and told me to see a surgeon in the morning about whether I would need skin grafts.*

*After arriving home, I tested and was told to keep the MAP coning open during the night. When I saw the doctor the next day, he was impressed at how well the burn looked. He said that it was well on its way to healing and would do so without any complications as long as we kept it clean. He also said that the wound would probably scab over in a few weeks, which would cause some pain and discomfort, but that would be normal.*

*He suggested that I get a tetanus shot. I do not like tetanus shots, but reasoned that it would be a good idea. Before getting the shot, I asked my MAP team to work with the tetanus and move whatever amount my body didn't need right on through. I encountered absolutely no pain or discomfort from this shot.*

*After the initial trauma passed, we began testing essences for different aspects of the wound—the large area that was burned, a smaller deeply bruised area, and two separate deep gashes. Each area required a different essence combination. I found that the flower essences that were needed for the deepest part of the wound related to the core issues that I have worked with healing throughout my life. As I healed physically, I found myself viewing my life differently, and was able to shift some very old limiting patterns. With this accident, I literally crashed and burned. Through feedback gained from the essences, I was able to rebuild my life in new and constructive ways.*

*All in all, I was told to keep the coning open for four straight days, which I did. Three days after the accident, I was able to travel on a plane for six hours. The wound healed without forming a scab. Within four weeks, I no longer needed to bandage the wound. And now, about four months later, there is just a faint scar to remind me of this MAP miracle. I am very thankful for the support that MAP and flower essences provided during this experience.*

S.J., Alaska

*Last summer, I seriously cut three fingers on my right hand while mowing the lawn. One was cut off completely at the top joint. As soon as it happened, I called for assistance from the Emergency MAP Team. I was told "Everything will be all right" and felt a deep calm. It was so reassuring that I had no problem driving myself to the hospital, and never went into shock.*

*When the doctor in the emergency room began surgery, I talked to the EMAT (Emergency Medical Assistance Team) again, and experienced the room flowing with a wonderful light energy. My friend holding my other hand and watching the surgery said a noticeable change came over the young and somewhat inexperienced doctor. His shaky hands became calm, and he smoothly stitched the fingertips of my three fingers back together. Throughout the surgery, I focused on bringing energy down through my crown to my heart. My friend was sending energy out into my right hand as it was being sutured. All the while, we both felt this tremendous loving presence that filled the room.*

*Now, seven months later, the fingers have healed nicely. I have had MAP sessions consistently throughout this period and have continued to ask for healing in these fingers. The doctor is extremely pleased at my progress. There are only a few things I can't do as well as I could before the injury, but these are also diminishing.*

*I am very grateful to the Emergency Medical Assistance Team and feel very blessed to have known about this magnificent assistance at that crucial time. I would like to see the word get out to all who are open to this valuable resource.*

P.D., Maryland

*Chapter 7*

# *Surrogating MAP For Children and Adults*

## MAP FOR CHILDREN: UPDATED

WHEN I WROTE THE FIRST EDITION of *MAP,* it was quite clear that the MAP teams wanted people to develop their personal relationship with the program before attempting to use it with children. After all, to work the program effectively with children, an adult must be present, supportive and comfortable with kinesiology and working with MAP.

Generally, children do not need the kind of intensive help that MAP offers. The majority of "normal" childhood health issues can be effectively helped with ETS Plus and essences.

However, if you have a child who has a chronic illness and the essence testing isn't working for you, or your child has a serious condition, is faced with an upcoming and potentially traumatic change, or has just gone through one, you might consider "putting" him or her into MAP.

To do this, you must be prepared to function as the child's support throughout the entire session. My first suggestion is that you do not attempt to activate MAP for a child until you have worked with the program yourself for *at least five months.*

● Your participation in children's MAP. You will need to remain with your child for the entire session and assist him throughout. For some sessions, you will just be sitting there the entire forty minutes quietly focused on your child and the session. That is, you will be passively present. During these times, you are to remain present (this is *not* free time for knitting or writing letters or drawing). The team needs to be able to get your attention if they need you to give ETS Plus to your child, if you are including this in the MAP sessions, or touch him in a specific way for either comfort or stabilization. At other times, you will be actively present. This means you get to jump into action. You will also have to know enough about the different sensations to be able to reassure and comfort your child if he becomes frightened. And you will need to be able to communicate with the MAP team, using either kinesiology or whatever other method you have developed with your team, in order to discern specifics that the team wishes to pass along as well as your child's session schedule.

● Communication. A child's MAP team talks to the parent, not to the child, about medical treatment and specifics. It is advisable to take notes during each session. Record the questions you ask and their answers; any insights you receive; any changes in diet; any changes in sleep or play activity. Ask the team the same kinds of comprehensive questions you would want to ask a good, communicative pediatrician.

In short, in a child's MAP session, the adult functions in the same responsible role as when taking the child to a pediatrician. The adult is actively present, gives pertinent information, asks questions and receives instructions from the pediatrician. The same things are done in a MAP session. In essence, you have to be confident enough about MAP to function as a competent, relaxed support person.

*Under no circumstances should you activate MAP for a child unless you can meet these criteria.*

● PERMISSION AND LEGAL GUARDIANSHIP. I would also like to point out that you should not activate MAP for a child unless you are the legal guardian of the child or have permission from that child's legal guardian. I don't mean to emphasize law here, but rather intent. Legal guardianship implies certain rights between an adult and a child that include the right to make this kind of decision for the child. When a child is young, the parents or guardians take responsibility for making all the decisions concerning that child's health care. This is an implied responsibility that goes along with the position. At a certain age—which is different for each child—the child begins to participate in these decisions. At whatever point you feel comfortable with the level of maturity of the child to have a say in his or her health care, this is also the time when a child is capable of saying whether they wish to participate in MAP.

● CHILDREN FLYING SOLO. There is the issue of when to allow your child to do MAP without an adult present. I've heard parents say, rather proudly, that their child is doing MAP by age seven or age nine, or whatever. (Always, of course, the child is "special" or "gifted.") It seems to me this becomes a point of pride or some kind of race with parents—like how early their child is potty trained, walking, speaking and reading. A MAP session is not about competition, nor is it a classroom or day-care center. It is a legitimate medical experience. If you don't think your child is mature enough to decide when he needs to see a doctor, and you don't feel comfortable letting him go through a doctor's appointment alone, assume that it is not appropriate to allow your child to schedule and go through a MAP session alone. Give your child and his MAP team the support that is needed so that the health issues can be properly addressed.

Luckily, the MAP teams aren't dumb. If they see that a child who is not capable of handling sessions alone yet has opened one without an adult present, the team will not get into any serious work with the child. So you don't have to panic around this issue and hide the MAP steps from him. Your child is safe. The team will stabilize and relax your child, then wait for him to close the coning. If your child just gets up and trundles on to another "toy," the team will automatically close the coning for him. (The teams do not give this "service" to adults. They feel it is important that a capable adult assume the responsibility for closing a MAP coning himself.)

● If your child becomes ill or is facing something else that is out of his usual pattern, and he has worked with a MAP team alone, don't assume it is appropriate for him to have sessions alone for this particular situation. If you are concerned and you want the team to work effectively and efficiently on your child, take the session seriously and be present for support and any needed assistance.

● Annoying your adult children. There is another age issue around MAP and children. We are all somebody's child. (Unless you are an alien and were formed from pond scum.) Here's the scenario: You are fifty-nine years old. You have been doing MAP for a year. You have found it to be an amazing and outstanding tool. It has given you the leg up on health issues you have struggled with for the last forty years. You have a forty-year-old son with asthma—and the idiot smokes on top of it. You know MAP could help him. But he thinks you are crazy and would not be open to anything like MAP. It's all alternative crap to him. *It is not ethical to try to sneak him into a MAP session without his conscious permission.* You may be his parent, but he is an adult, and his rights supersede yours. You do not have the right, even as his parent, to interfere in this way. A MAP team will not participate in a sneak attack, no matter how well intentioned a parent may be.

● EMOTIONAL HEALTH SESSIONS FOR CHILDREN. There is one area of health where it is appropriate for a child to develop a personal, private relationship with their MAP team. This is the area of emotional health. Think. Normally it is not appropriate for a parent to be present during a child's session with his or her therapist or counselor. The same would be true in MAP. If a child is comfortable with MAP and wishes for such a therapeutic situation, some place to go to share his thoughts, pain, anger, fear and sadness, this is an excellent solution. In this situation, it would be best if the child knew how to open and close the coning and take ETS Plus.

If your child feels more comfortable with you opening and closing the coning, you may do so. Open a regular child's MAP coning (including your higher self), then leave the room to give your child privacy. After the forty-minute session, return and close the coning. Then administer the three doses of ETS Plus as outlined. Your child needs you to open and close the coning—therefore your higher self is an essential part of the coning. Your presence in the coning is reassuring and comforting—and is still needed.

## MAP STEPS FOR CHILDREN

### The Scanning Session: Updated

1 OPEN THE CONING. The following is the coning for the children's MAP scanning session:

- Overlighting Deva of Healing (Wait ten seconds.)
- Pan (Wait ten seconds.)
- White Brotherhood Medical Unit (Wait ten seconds.)
- Your higher self (Wait ten seconds.)
- The child's higher self (Wait ten seconds.)

Wait another ten to fifteen seconds for you and your child to adjust to the coning. Optional: Both of you take ETS Plus.

● SETUP. Inform the White Brotherhood that you are acting on behalf of this child.

● THE SLEEPING CHILD. Your child can be asleep for the scanning session. You may prefer this since it is easier to keep a sleeping child still! If possible, it would be best for the child to be lying on his back. But if this is not possible, the team will work around it. Do not hold your child in your arms or on your lap for the session.

If your child is asleep and is too old to be given ETS Plus on the forehead (see p. 168), just take a dose of ETS Plus for yourself after opening the coning. If your child is awake, give him his dose of ETS Plus (ten to twelve drops). By taking ETS Plus yourself, you are ensuring that you are fully stabilized in the coning. However, the MAP teams do not want you to wake your child for his dose because the advantages to both the team and the parent of working with a sleeping child are so great.

2 THE SCANNING. Placing your two hands side by side, palms down and parallel to the reclining child about three inches above the body, "scan" the child's body system to the team. (See the drawing on p. 162.) This differentiates your body energy from the child's and connects the team with the child's system. Do this by moving your hands in concert, starting from the top or crown of the head, and moving slowly down the body to the bottoms of the feet. As you move down the trunk, move your hands in concert to scan each arm and then each leg. The movement should be slow and steady, and the scanning should take about ten minutes. If you can "hear" the team, they may tell you to hold the scanning at certain spots. Just stop your hands and hold them above the child's body until you get the go-ahead to start moving your hands again.

3 SESSION TIME AND CODE. The scanning session will last one hour. For this session, you do not need to verbalize any problems or issues your child is dealing with. This is a quiet session for you. At the end of the hour, *you* request that you be given your child's team code. You will use this code to open any future sessions for your child. If and when your child takes over his own sessions, he will also use this code.

4 CLOSE DOWN THE SESSION exactly as you would for yourself, only now you must disconnect your higher self *and* the child's higher self. (See p. 176, step 3.)

5 ETS PLUS. Take one dose of ETS Plus for yourself right after closing the coning, just in case your being in the coning threw your balance off. Then give your child *one dose* of ETS Plus to help stabilize him after his first experience in a MAP coning. However, if you're not using ETS Plus, your child

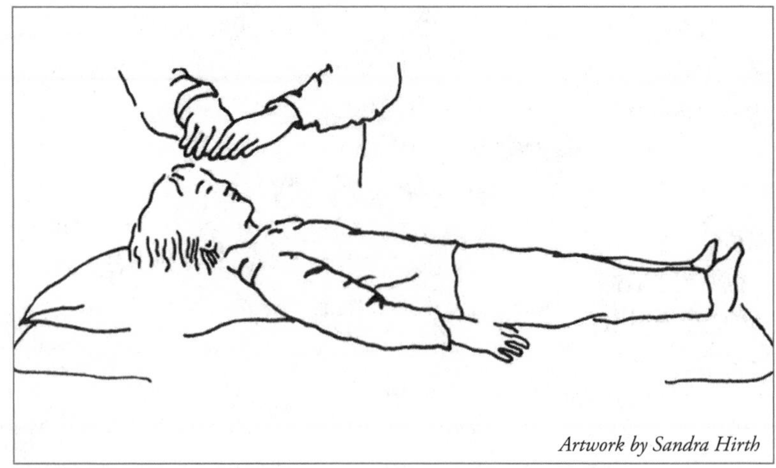

*Artwork by Sandra Hirth*

will be fine. It's an option. (See p. 168.) Make sure the child spends a few moments quietly before going on about his day. Wait twenty-four hours before opening the next session.

## Regular MAP Sessions for Children: Updated

Most parents prefer for their child to be asleep for regular MAP sessions. Try to position them on their back, if possible. If not, the team will work around the contortions, but they won't be able to work quite as efficiently. Recommended: ETS Plus.

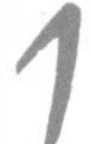

1 OPEN A CHILDREN'S MAP CONING using your child's team code. The children's MAP coning includes:

- Overlighting Deva of Healing
- Pan
- White Brotherhood Medical Team (visualize team code)
- Your higher self
- Your child's higher self

Wait ten to fifteen seconds.

● Take one dose of ETS Plus for yourself. If your child is awake, give him one dose of ETS Plus. This ensures you both are stabilized in the coning. However, don't wake your child to give him his dose of ETS Plus. A sleeping child is a major plus.

2 THE SESSION. The regular sessions for a child are also forty minutes. Tell the team all the information you can think of about your child's health patterns and problems—physical, emotional, mental and spiritual. Be as comprehensive about your child as you are with your own team. It might be helpful to write down specific points you don't want to forget before going into the session.

● At the end of forty minutes, ask for any information about treatment or changes. Then find out from the team when they wish to work with your child again. It won't be like the adult schedule. It will be less frequent, unless there is a chronic, serious problem. I am not giving a prescribed schedule of sessions for children as I did for adults because it is assumed that any adult participating in a child's session will be able to communicate with the team. This way, they will be able to get the schedule that is best for their child.

● HINT: It is easier to keep your focus if you say something out loud. However, this does not mean you have to say it so loud that you will wake your child. Whispering is fine.

3 CLOSE DOWN THE CONING and take one dose of ETS Plus for yourself. (See p. 177.)

4 ETS PLUS FOR YOUR CHILD. Recommended. (See p. 168.) You will need to wake your child and administer *three doses* of ETS Plus. Give him the first dose immediately after closing the coning. Wait five minutes, then give him the second dose. Wait five more minutes and give him the final dose.

## ADDITIONAL INFORMATION

● Touching and holding your child. It is important that you not hold your child during the session because the mixing of the two sets of energy will be too much for the team to separate and discern well. However, if you must touch your child during the session or hold him if he should become frightened, you may do so. The team will stop the session until you are finished. The forty minutes does not include "comfort breaks." So be aware of how much time is taken and add this to the forty minutes.

● Touching and holding upon request. Sometimes the team will ask you to touch or hold your child in a specific way. This stabilizes him during the session. The most common "hold" involves placing one hand under the back of the neck (the cervicals) and the other hand at the very base or bottom of the back, just at the tailbone. This hand is stabilizing the sacrum. They may request that you hold your hands in this position anywhere from five to twenty minutes. They don't want you to lift the child up to do this. They just want you to place or slide your hands to these two areas and hold them there. Also you may feel intuitively that you are to touch or hold something. Before jumping into action, check your intuition with the team, either verbally or with kinesiology. Make sure you understand where they want you to hold.

● Keeping good notes. As I've already mentioned, be sure to keep good notes on all the questions asked in a session, any insights or information you are given by the team, session scheduling. . . . You'll be referring back to the notes a lot. Also, keep notes of questions you think about and want to ask in the next session.

● ASKING QUESTIONS. Ask lots of questions, and don't be afraid to make them practical. Focus on what is needed to get your child through the illness or injury as efficiently and effectively as possible. If your child is sick, don't waste time by asking a bunch of questions about whether this is some karmic holdover from your child's lifetime as an alcoholic ice sculptor in ancient Iceland. If something like this is important, you'll get the insight from the team. You don't have to go digging for it. Instead, ask about diet, flower essences, number of days of bed rest needed, and anything else that's immediately practical and helpful that you can think of.

● COMBINING CHILDREN'S MAP WITH OTHER TREATMENTS. As with adults, MAP is not opposed to your using over-the-counter medicines or prescription drugs, seeing doctors or going to the hospital for children. Sometimes working from both ends of the situation is the most efficient route. They may suggest something to you along these lines. If you aren't confident about hearing them, ask direct questions about the regular medical assistance that is available to you. And even if the team says a doctor's visit is not needed but you feel uncomfortable about this, then take the child to the doctor. Do what you need to do to feel comfortable and what you feel is best for your child.

● MAP AND DOCTOR'S VISITS. When you take your child to the doctor, open the coning for his team and keep the coning open throughout the visit. This gives the team the information they need to appropriately support and assist what is happening. After the visit, ask the team when they would like their next "appointment" with your child, then close the coning and administer ETS Plus as you would for a Regular Children's MAP session.

● FOLLOW-UP SESSION SCHEDULE. As the supporting adult, you will need to take responsibility for getting the schedule for any follow-up sessions and letting the team know during these sessions any changes you have observed in your child's condition or pattern of behavior. Include both positive and difficult changes. This lets the team know how your child is integrating their work. You will need to do follow-up sessions for your child just as you would for yourself.

● CHILDREN'S MAP ISN'T FOR EVERY CHILD. Do not put a child into MAP if that child is frightened of a concept like MAP or is easily frightened by life. This is not the program for that child, no matter how much MAP could help. It would be unfair and unnecessarily frightening for such a child to deal with MAP. Use flower essences in this case.

● DO NOT DISTURB! Some parents who regularly use MAP with their children have said to me that sometimes they will open the coning while their child is asleep but they "hear" or feel strongly that the child does not wish to be disturbed. Even though the child is asleep, his higher self knows you just opened a MAP coning. Apparently this kid doesn't want a session right then or is busy. Do not override this. The parents who have talked about it say it is unmistakable—and often funny. They just say quietly "okay" and close the session. Sometime during the next night or two, they try again—and everything is fine. There's no resistance.

● MAP BEFORE THEY'RE SICK. If you wish to incorporate MAP in your child's health care program, do the scanning session and several regular sessions with your child as soon as possible to get the team set up and to get you comfortable with working with the team. Don't wait for your child to get sick before doing this.

● MAP COMBINED WITH OTHER PERELANDRA PROCESSES. If your child needs a process like the Perelandra Body/Soul Fusion Process, plan to do it while he is in a MAP session. This allows the team to support and assist your child as he moves through the process. Open the session, state your intention of doing the process, verify with the team that it is a good time to do the process, and then move through the steps as outlined. Doing it in MAP does not alter any of the process steps. (The Body/Soul Fusion Process is explained in Perelandra Paper #4. Our contact information is in the back of this book.)

## MAP/Calibration for Children

You would use the MAP/Calibration combination for a child in the same kinds of situations you would use it for yourself. Consider a MAP/Calibration session when your child is mentally or emotionally stuck, unable to move forward, or suffering from learning disabilities. First, however, try working with these problems by using flower essences. Really, the vast majority of these kinds of issues can be easily addressed with the essences. Children often respond to flower essences far more strongly and easily than adults. And essence testing is less time consuming than MAP or MAP/Calibration sessions. So, first try several essence dosages.

If you have questions about whether a specific problem should be addressed with essences or with MAP or MAP/Calibration, you can open a MAP coning with your child's team (without your child being present) and ask the questions. It is essentially like a consultation call.

### Administering ETS Plus to Children

I strongly suggest you include it, especially when working with children and MAP. There is no learning curve and no testing involved. In short, it's too easy to use ETS Plus to not include it, and its benefits in stabilizing and supporting the MAP work are exceptional.

● Topical and oral applications. For children from birth to four years old who are asleep, ETS Plus can be administered on the forehead. The teams can assist its absorption into the electrical system for a child up to age four. Over age four, you may skip the dose usually given after the coning is first opened if your child is sleeping. But you will need to wake him up once the coning is closed and give him the three doses of ETS Plus as outlined. You can cut the alcohol- or vinegar-preservative taste by diluting the ETS Plus drops in a little bit of water—no more than a quarter of a cup. But your child will need to take all of this solution at one time. He may not sip it over a period of time.

## LASSIE TO THE RESCUE

Oh, yes... here's one more piece of information about MAP teams for children. When Children's MAP first began, several of the teams included a big, overly lovable, huggable dog. She didn't function in a medical capacity (just in case you were wondering), but the teams found that her presence was calming to some children. Often, children saw her or felt her hot breath panting over them. Sometimes, even the parents saw her or felt that breath. And they said that their child visibly relaxed when she was around. Because she has been such a help, the MAP teams have expanded on this idea over the years and have established a Children's MAP Canine Corps. So, if your child talks about a dog on the team, that's not his imagination running rampant!

## SURROGATING MAP FOR ADULTS

Let's get real here. MAP is a very simple process. If a person is too ill or injured to activate and participate in sessions on their own, and they would like MAP's help, you can help them by using the Emergency MAP Procedure. Other than this, there's really no need to surrogate MAP for an adult. It is very important that an adult interested in MAP really wants it enough to initiate it. This program has to hit a person in their heart, soul and gut. If someone who is perfectly capable of following the simple MAP steps is asking you to surrogate them for you, it is probably a sign that they really don't want to be in the program. They are hesitating and they need more time. The MAP steps could not be easier, but the program itself takes time, effort, intent and diligence on the person's part. They need to be wholeheartedly committed. If they are hesitating, encourage them to back off, and let them know that backing off is really okay.

● HELPING SOMEONE TO GET STARTED. The best way to help someone get into MAP is to spend time going over the steps with them. Tell them how easy it is to open a coning. Talk to them about your experiences in opening a coning. Show them kinesiology and work with them on it. Talk about ETS Plus. And talk about your MAP experiences. But don't just leave it at that. Either loan the person your copy of the book *MAP* or get another copy for them. Don't let them jump into the program with just your understanding of the steps and your experiences. Be sure they have the book with all the steps as they are to be followed and the more complete information about the program itself for reference.

● EXCEPTION TO THE RULE. There is one exception to the "Don't Surrogate for Adults" rule. If you are the legal guardian of a mentally or emotionally challenged adult who can not work with MAP on their own but you feel would be comfortable in the program, you may function as their MAP surrogate. In this case, set up according to the steps for Children's MAP. You will function in the support capacity as outlined in those steps.

*Chapter 8*

# *Quick Reference Steps*

## FIRST SESSION: THE SCANNING SESSION

Have ETS Plus (optional), a clock, paper and pen handy.

1 Open the coning. Wait 10 seconds after each connection. State:

*I'd like to open a MAP coning. I'd like to connect with:*

- *the Overlighting Deva of Healing,*
- *Pan,*
- *the White Brotherhood Medical Unit,*
- *my higher self.*

Wait another 10–15 seconds.

2 During the scanning session, you do not need to talk. Remain still for one hour. At the end of the hour, request that you be given your team's code.

3 Close the coning. *I'd like to disconnect from:*

- *my higher self,*
- *the White Brotherhood Medical Unit and my team,*
- *Pan,*
- *the Overlighting Deva of Healing.*

Wait 10–15 seconds. Optional: Take one dose of ETS Plus. Record your team code. Wait 24 hours before the second session.

## REGULAR SESSIONS

Have ETS Plus (optional), a clock, paper and pen handy.

1 Open a MAP coning:

- Overlighting Deva of Healing
- Pan
- White Brotherhood Medical Team
  (Visualize or say your team's identification code.)
- Your higher self

Wait 10–15 seconds. Optional: Take one dose of ETS Plus.

2 Describe *fully* how you are feeling. Tell your team everything that comes to mind. Give feedback on any sensations, pleasant or difficult, that you feel during the session. Optional: Take ETS Plus should you feel discomfort.
The session lasts 40 minutes.

3 At the end of 40 minutes, thank your team and close the coning:

- Your higher self
- White Brotherhood Medical Team
- Pan
- Overlighting Deva of Healing

Once the coning is closed, wait 10–15 seconds.

4 Optional: Take three doses of ETS Plus to stabilize the session. Take the first dose immediately after closing down the coning. Wait five minutes, then take the second dose. Wait five more minutes and take the final dose.

Spend a few minutes quietly before continuing with your day.

## MAP/CALIBRATION SESSIONS

Have ETS Plus (required), a clock, paper and pen handy.

1 Open the MAP session as usual:

- Overlighting Deva of Healing
- Pan
- White Brotherhood Medical Team
  (Visualize or say your team's identification code.)
- Your higher self

Wait 10–15 seconds. Take one dose of ETS Plus.

2 When you wish to switch to the Calibration Process, state:

*I'd like to set up for a MAP/Calibration, and I'd like to shift Pan forward.*

Wait 5 to 10 seconds for this connection and shift.

3 Describe your difficulty or issue, giving as much information about it as possible. The Calibration lasts 30 minutes.

4 At the end of the 30 minutes, end the Calibration Process and shift back to the regular MAP coning. To do this, state:

*I'd like to close the Calibration, and I'd like to shift Pan back into the MAP focus.*

Wait 5 seconds. Take one dose of ETS Plus.

5 Complete your regular MAP session. Make sure you spend a total of forty minutes for MAP plus the thirty minutes for the Calibration.

6 When the MAP session is complete, close down the coning as you normally would. (See p. 172, step 3.) Wait 10–15 seconds.

7 *Required:* Take three doses of ETS Plus to stabilize the session. Take the first dose immediately after closing down the coning. Wait five minutes, then take the second dose. Wait five more minutes and take the final dose. Spend a few minutes quietly before continuing with your day.

## EMERGENCY MAP PROCEDURE

1 Open the coning by stating:
*I want to open an Emergency MAP coning with the _________ team.*
(Insert your team's identification code.)

2 Recommended: Take one dose of ETS Plus every 3 to 5 minutes for the first 20 minutes.

3 Recommended: After the 20 minutes, take one dose of ETS Plus every 30 to 40 minutes for the next 2 to 3 hours.

4 Stay connected with the Emergency MAP coning and team throughout the time it takes you to stabilize from the emergency, including any hospitalization. Recommended: Take ETS Plus four times daily throughout this period.

5 Once stabilized (or at home), get a follow-up MAP schedule and close the Emergency MAP coning. State:
*I'd like to close the Emergency MAP coning.*
Recommended: Take one dose of ETS Plus after closing.

## SURROGATING EMERGENCY MAP

1 ● TO OPEN THE CONING FOR SOMEONE ALREADY USING MAP. State:

*I request that an Emergency MAP coning be opened and that _________ (person) be connected to his/her team.* (State or visualize the person's team code or name of the person, if you don't know the code.)

● TO OPEN A CONING FOR SOMEONE WHO DOES NOT HAVE A MAP TEAM.

- Get conscious permission to open an Emergency MAP coning.
- Once permission is granted, open the coning. State:
  *I want to open an Emergency MAP coning for _________.* (Insert name of person in trouble.)

2 Recommended: Administer ETS Plus to him every 3 to 5 minutes for the first 20 minutes.

3 Recommended: After the 20 minutes, continue giving one dose of ETS Plus every 30 to 40 minutes for the next 2 to 3 hours.

4 Once the person is stabilized (or at home), close the Emergency MAP coning. State:

*I request that _________'s Emergency MAP coning now be closed.*

Recommended: Administer one dose of ETS Plus. If he wishes to get into MAP on his own, give him the book and help him understand the steps.

## CHILDREN'S SCANNING SESSION

Have ETS Plus (optional), a clock, paper and pen handy.

1 Open a children's MAP coning:
(Wait 10 seconds after each connection.)

- Overlighting Deva of Healing
- Pan
- White Brotherhood Medical Unit
- Your higher self
- The child's higher self

Wait another 10–15 seconds. Optional: Take ETS Plus and administer one dose to your child.

SET UP. Inform the White Brotherhood Medical Unit that you are acting on behalf of this child.

2 Scan the child with both hands. The scanning session lasts one hour. At the end, ask for the child's team code. Record the team's identification code.

3 Close the coning:

- The child's higher self
- Your higher self
- White Brotherhood Medical Unit and child's team
- Pan
- Overlighting Deva of Healing

Wait another 10–15 seconds. Optional: Immediately after closing the coning, take one dose of ETS Plus and administer one dose to your child.

## CHILDREN'S REGULAR SESSIONS

Have ETS Plus (recommended), a clock, paper/pen handy.

1 Open the children's MAP coning using your child's team code:

- Overlighting Deva of Healing
- Pan
- White Brotherhood Medical Team
  (Visualize or say your child's team code.)
- Your higher self
- The child's higher self

Wait 10–15 seconds. Recommended: Take one dose of ETS Plus and administer one dose to your child.

2 Regular sessions last 40 minutes. Tell the team the state of your child's health. Be prepared to assist and offer support. Take notes. Ask questions. Get any prescribed treatments or changes.

3 Close the coning:

- The child's higher self
- Your higher self
- White Brotherhood Medical Team
- Pan
- Overlighting Deva of Healing

Wait another 10–15 seconds.

Recommended: Take one dose of ETS Plus. Administer three doses of ETS Plus to your child to stabilize the MAP work. Give her the first dose immediately after closing down the coning. Wait five minutes, then give her the second dose. Wait five more minutes and give her the final dose.

## SURROGATING MAP FOR ADULTS

1 Don't. In an emergency, follow the Surrogating Emergency MAP steps. (See p. 175.)

## OPENING A PROFESSIONAL MAP TEAM

1 Make sure you have a comfortable and confident relationship with your personal MAP team.

Have ETS Plus (optional), a clock, paper and pen handy. (Read chapter 9 before using these Quick Reference steps.)

2 Open the following MAP coning:

- Overlighting Deva of Healing
- Pan
- White Brotherhood Medical Unit
- Your higher self

Wait 10–15 seconds. Optional: Take one dose of ETS Plus.

3 State: *I want to work with a Professional MAP team to shift my practice to the new medical dynamics.*
Describe the health care area you work in.

4 Request a professional team code. Record the code.

5 Get acquainted. Ask pertinent questions regarding your schedule for setting up Professional MAP team meetings. Schedule one or more monitoring sessions when you will be working with clients.

6 Close the coning:
- Your higher self
- White Brotherhood Medical Unit and Your Professional MAP Team
- Pan
- Overlighting Deva of Healing

Once the coning is closed, wait 10–15 seconds.
Optional: Take one dose of ETS Plus.

## REGULAR PROFESSIONAL MAP SESSIONS

1 Open a Professional MAP coning using your professional team's identification code.
- Overlighting Deva of Healing
- Pan
- Your Professional MAP Team (Visualize or say your team's identification code.)
- Your higher self

Wait 10–15 seconds. Take one dose of ETS Plus.

2 If you are seeing clients, go about your day, but be aware of any assistance your team might be offering.

3 After the last client, close down the coning. Take another dose of ETS Plus.

● TEAM MEETINGS. For meetings in which you plan to work with your team outside client visits, open your Professional MAP Team coning. Take ETS Plus. Have your meeting for however long you wish.

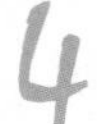 When your meeting is finished, close the coning:

- Your higher self
- Your Professional MAP Team
- Pan
- Overlighting Deva of Healing

Once the coning is closed, wait 10–15 seconds. Then take one dose of ETS Plus.

*Chapter 9*

# *Professional MAP Teams*

WE ARE PRESENTLY INVOLVED in the transition from the Piscean to the Aquarian era. This shift requires us to develop a new intellectual outlook and new ways of working with and within the Aquarian dynamic. *Everything* is moving through this transition. This includes our physical body. Even on a cellular level we are now responding to the new, and moving away from the old.

This change has created an ever-widening gap in our health care systems. To be effective during the Piscean era, our allopathic and alternative modalities had to address healing balance within the Piscean dynamic. What we have now are allopathic and alternative health systems that address balance from the Piscean perspective. At the same time, we have a growing number of people who are altering the balance and rhythm of their bodies and lifestyles in response to the new Aquarian dynamic. This has created a gap in health care. Systems and modalities that worked well a few years ago are less effective today. Some health care practitioners recognize this and are trying mightily to address it. But for the most part, they are operating on a wing and a prayer and with good intentions—hoping what they are doing differently will be helpful.

In order to be effective, all health care practices must now correspond to the Aquarian transition dynamic. Old definitions, approaches and expectations must be replaced with new ways of thinking and functioning.

Working with a Professional MAP team is the most effective way to make these changes because the White Brotherhood Medical Unit and nature fully understand the new era we are moving into and what changes we have to make during the transition. They have the knowledge, understanding and ability to create structures that support us through the transition. And—equally important—they are eager to work with us in a professional capacity to do just this if we consciously request their assistance.

If you are a health care practitioner and want to include the new Aquarian health and healing dynamics in your practice, you may work with a Professional MAP team. This team is different from your personal MAP team because its focus will be the direction and nature of your professional work.

Here's what you do:

1 You must establish a *personal* MAP team and move through the initial five-month program outlined in this book. Besides stabilizing and balancing your health, this will give you ample time to learn to work with MAP.

2 After the five months, if you would like to work with a Professional MAP team but you are not yet confident or comfortable working with your personal team, take more time to gain this confidence and comfort. Take all the time you need. The critical issue is the development of your ability to communicate effectively with your team and your physical

ability to function within a coning for a specific period of time. You will not be able to work with a Professional MAP team unless you can communicate with them (using kinesiology is fine) and work in the coning for long periods of time. So, the time you spend developing your ability to stabilize physically while in a coning and developing the different skills in your working relationship with your personal team builds the foundation you need to work with the professional team.

Once you are comfortable working with your personal team, open the following MAP coning (you are *not* connected to your personal MAP team when doing this):

- Overlighting Deva of Healing
- Pan
- White Brotherhood Medical Unit
- Your higher self

Take one dose of ETS Plus.... If this sounds familiar it is because this is how you opened the first coning for the scanning session with MAP.

3 Tell this group that you want to work with a Professional MAP team to shift your practice to the new medical dynamics. Then describe the area of health care you work in. By the time you have finished defining or describing your work, you will be connected to your Professional MAP team. It will be comprised of members of the White Brotherhood Medical Unit who work specifically in your area.

4 Request a professional team code. You will now have two codes. One you will use when connecting with your personal team, and the other you will use when connecting with your professional team. *When you work with a professional*

*team, you do not drop your personal team.* The professional team works solely with you in the development and implementation of the new dynamics in your health care practice. It also works with you as the practitioner. Your personal team will continue to work with you for illnesses, imbalances, personal emotional processes and other areas of personal growth. You will continue addressing the same kinds of issues with your personal team as you did prior to opening a MAP professional team.

5 Begin to get acquainted. Ask questions you have regarding working together. Ask if they have suggestions for you about setting up your working relationship. Use this session to lay as much of the groundwork for working together as you can. Ask about how often you should meet and time limits for the working sessions.

NOTE: They may want you to wait until after the monitoring session (explained in the paragraph below) to work out the meeting schedule. Ask the team if they would like to wait before discussing a session schedule. If you communicate using kinesiology, word your questions in the simple yes/no format.

● THE MONITORING SESSION. They will want to monitor you at work before giving you any work-related suggestions, and possibly prior to setting up a meeting schedule, so plan a time with them when they can do this monitoring session.

For the monitoring, all you need to do is open your Professional MAP team coning (using their code) prior to seeing a client. (You do not need to do this in front of the client. The team will be monitoring your work and how the client responds. It will not be working personally with the client. Therefore, no permission is needed from the client.) The team will take it from there. After the client leaves, you can either close the coning, leave it open for a second client monitoring, or have a question-and-answer session with your team about any changes they might suggest in your approach based on what they have already seen. If they were only able to monitor your work with one client, ask your team if they would like to monitor additional clients. If they do, ask how many more clients the team would like to monitor, and have those sessions as soon as possible. (If using kinesiology, you get this information by doing sequential testing. This is explained in Appendix B, p. 245.)

6 When working with the professional team during regular office sessions, you will open the coning at the beginning of your workday. You must remember to close the coning at the end of each day when you are finished working—*do not leave it open all night.* An open coning such as this will unnecessarily drain your energy and you will feel dog tired.

● PHYSICALLY SUPPORTING THIS WORK. Pay attention to your energy level when you first begin to work with your Professional MAP team. You may be able to keep the coning open easily for half your day or a quarter of your day. But if you try to keep the coning open for the entire day, you might feel drained. This is because your "muscles" are not yet fully conditioned. So, work with the coning in the beginning only as long as you are physically capable. If you are not clear about the state of your "conditioning," ask your professional team how long they recommend you work in an activated coning in the beginning. In time, your conditioning will strengthen, and you will easily be able to keep the coning open for the full workday.

NOTE: Take one dose of ETS Plus every day just after opening and closing that coning. This will help balance you while you work in the coning. And, if after a while you feel your conditioning is not strengthening, ask your team what you need to do to assist this process. You may need a diet change or more sleep—something simple such as this.

● YOUR TEAM'S ROLE IN PROFESSIONAL MAP. When working with a client with an open Professional MAP coning, your team will be observing you in your role as physician or practitioner. The team does not work on the client. As you work, you may receive ideas, intuitive hits and verbal suggestions from your team about more effective ways you can achieve your goals with this client. To facilitate the process, you may choose to include the client's higher self in the coning during his appointment. This allows your team a greater depth and range of what it can suggest to you as it observes your interaction with that client on all levels.

● THE CONING AND THE CLIENT'S HIGHER SELF. The MAP teams do not want your client's higher self in the coning while he is being worked on, *unless he has given his conscious consent* to be included in the coning. As I have already stated, the MAP team is working with the practitioner and is not the client's personal team. To obtain conscious consent you have to explain to your client that you are working in a new manner and with a different kind of team, and give him a general idea of what is involved with a coning. You do not have to explain MAP since the team will not be working directly with the client. Once he has a basic understanding of a coning and how you are working, he can decide whether he wants his higher self in the coning.

*When the appointment is over, and before your client leaves your office, you must disconnect his higher self from the coning. Do not work with another client with someone else's higher self in the coning.*

● CONNECTING/DISCONNECTING THE CLIENT'S HIGHER SELF. To include a client's higher self in the MAP coning, just state that you'd like the person's higher self included in the opened coning. This will occur immediately. To disconnect that higher self, state that you'd like it to be disconnected from the coning. The coning can be modified in this manner every time you include someone's higher self. You do not have to open a coning from scratch or close the whole thing down if all you want to do is either add or subtract a client's higher self from that coning.

It would be good to give your client a dose of ETS Plus just after including him in the coning and again after disconnecting him from the coning. This way you can ensure the client is fully stabilized during and after the coning experience.

● INFORMING CLIENTS OF THE CHANGE. The Professional MAP teams recommend that when you expand your practice to include them you inform your clients that you are changing how you work. Let them know that they may observe differences and that they should give you as much feedback as possible about differences they perceive in themselves. It would be helpful to assure your clients that you are available to them if they need to call. Some of their reactions to the new work may be dramatic and unexpected, and additional support from you would be appreciated. Let them know you are moving into something new and that you want them to feel comfortable with it and participate as much as possible.

● CREATING AN EFFECTIVE TEAM. Opening a Professional MAP team is easy. What is challenging is establishing a good, effective, working relationship. One thing you will feel right away is your team's eagerness to work with you professionally and support you as you go through the changes needed to work with them. To create an effective team, you must understand that *you* are a partner. Your team will be working with you in two ways:

- while you work with clients;
- during private meetings with your team to work out changes and new approaches, discuss the physical setup and changes needed in your office space, and discuss issues with how you are working with specific clients. Remember, this team works with you professionally and not on you personally.

Get into a rhythm with your team. Open the coning whenever you are with a client, and then meet with your team regularly for additional input, change and insight. You can ask your team how often you should meet with them.

● PRACTICE PATIENCE. Sometimes you may ask your team for insight or understanding about a new procedure or result, and feel that they really don't want to answer your questions. If you "hear" your team, you can literally hear them back off from the questions. This is because you need to observe what's going on for a while before you can understand the answer to the questions. When we work in new areas, we sometimes don't understand what is going on because our understanding is based on logic built around old ways of doing things. So, if you sense them saying "Not yet," take the hint. You may need to observe something for a week, a month, even a year before you are able to understand answers to your questions.

● KEEP GOOD NOTES. This is not a suggestion; it is a requirement. Keep good notes. Keep notes about changes in your work, responses and reactions of clients, and information you get from your team during meetings. The biggest surprise shared by nearly every practitioner who is working with a Professional MAP team is the massive amount of information and insights they (the practitioner) are suddenly faced with. This is like entering medical school. And not only will you need to keep good notes, you will have to organize them. Either keep them on computer or in a loose-leaf notebook to allow you to separate and shift blocks of notes around. You will want to refer back to these notes. Although this sounds tedious and time consuming, trying to find a specific piece of information from a 400-page stack of scribbled notes that have no sense of organization about them is a horror show. Believe it or not, the record keeping is the thing that most often breaks the back of the aspiring Professional MAP team participant. So, right from the beginning, spend time thinking about how you want to set up this note-keeping business. Make it easy, convenient and super organized. Then once you figure out what you'd like, buy the stuff you need and use it.

If your carefully planned record-keeping system isn't working the way you had hoped it would, *quickly* modify what you've set up. The Professional MAP program isn't something that lasts for a week or a month. It is a long-term program. So keep working on this until you find the record-keeping system that is best for you.

● THE NOTES HELP ANCHOR YOU. Good notes organize your experience internally and externally. A lot will be happening and it will be helpful to keep a chronology of the changes, reactions and information. You will also want to refer to your notes when you realize your perception wasn't accurate. Knowing how you perceived what the team said will help you correct the error and understand how you got it wrong. That way you learn from mistakes and continue fine-tuning your working relationship with your team.

● ADJUSTING YOUR OFFICE PROCEDURES. It is easy to work with your team around such issues as how to change existing procedures if you organize your information. For example, let's say the team wants you to alter your basic office procedure. You got this by asking about the office procedure in a series of yes/no questions and using kinesiology. Suddenly you are faced with a large block of information—your entire office procedure—and you haven't a clue about how to change it.

1 Open your Professional MAP team coning, and list your office procedure step by step, starting from the moment the person walks in the door. Number each step—and don't include two steps together.

2 Then, with your team, go down the list, read each step, and ask if that step is to be changed. If you get a yes, check the step. You'll most likely find your entire procedure does not have to be changed, but just a few steps.

3 Focus on each step needing change and ask the team to give you insight about the change. Tell them what comes to mind and then test to see if your perception is accurate. Work with them on each step until you verify that you fully understand the changes.

4 When you have finished, read your new procedure step by step, testing each step as you go along. ("Is this step now complete?") If you get a negative response, this means that step needs to be further modified. Keep doing this until all the steps test positive.

One of the keys to working with your team is good information management, and modifying your office procedure is a good example of this. Whenever you are dealing with a large block of information, just break it down into simple, manageable pieces and work with one small piece at a time.

Start working with your team in a way that you feel is comfortable and reasonable. Don't feel you have to change how you work with all your clients right away. Do it in manageable increments and with clients with whom you feel most comfortable about making changes.

## THE PROFESSIONAL MAP CONING AND TIME MANAGEMENT

You don't want to remain in a Professional MAP coning longer than necessary. If you have one client scheduled in the morning and three clients scheduled in late afternoon, open the coning for the early client and then close the coning until the start of the afternoon sessions.

For days when clients are scheduled back to back, open the coning for the first client and leave it open throughout the day until the last client leaves. Then close the coning. It takes more effort and energy to open a coning than to sustain it. So you don't want to keep opening and closing conings throughout a day. However, you also don't want to expend energy to sustain the coning for unnecessarily long periods of time. You're going to have to use your judgment here. Your Professional MAP team can help you reach a balance if you are having trouble.

- LUNCH BREAKS. If you have the coning open all day, you don't need to keep it "active" during long breaks such as lunch. You can put a coning in an "at-rest" position simply by letting your team know you're going to lunch now (or whatever) and you'd like them to move into the at-rest position. You will feel an immediate easing within you. This way, you leave the coning open while expending very little energy to sustain it. After lunch, when you are getting ready for the next client, just tell the coning you're ready to work again, and you will feel an activation as they respond, if you feel such things.

- THEY ARE THERE FOR YOU. You can ask your Professional MAP team any question at any time while the coning is open and fully activated—that is, not in an "at-rest" position. You don't have to do any kind of preparation to talk with them. Once the coning is open, they are with you at all times.

- PROTEIN DRAIN. Working in a coning for long periods of time may cause a protein drain. Be aware of how you feel, and increase your protein intake on the days you are working with your Professional MAP team.

## WHAT TO EXPECT WHEN WORKING WITH A PROFESSIONAL MAP TEAM

● EXPECT VERY DIFFERENT RESULTS than you are used to. For example, herbologists using kinesiology will get different results that will make little, if any, sense regarding which herbs to use. If you are working in a system that has an established tradition of how elements such as herbs are used and what they work with, you have to disregard this information and allow new information to form.

● THE UNUSUAL AND STRONG. Expect different, sometimes unusual and sometimes strong responses and reactions to your work. MAP works in a more profound and comprehensive manner than you are used to. Your clients may have deeper and different responses than they formerly had. And the results can come more quickly than you are used to. You'll probably notice that your clients are more responsive to the new work.

Because of this, it is important that you offer support to your clients beyond the office. You may be pleasantly surprised at what you see happening, but your client might be frightened at the suddenness and intensity.

● INTUITIVE HITS. You will get strong intuitive "hits" regarding what you are doing with a client. Learn to go with these hits. This is one way your team works with you. If you are questioning the hit, verify it with your team prior to doing anything. Quietly ask if what you are perceiving is correct, then describe what you are perceiving and either listen for their answer or test using kinesiology.

● EXPECT THE SESSION TO MOVE DIFFERENTLY. You will feel your team help as you move along. Be prepared to change how you function in a session. You may receive a strong urging to do something you would not normally consider. In these cases, trust your intuition and just do it. The proof of its accuracy will be in the results.

● GIVE THE TEAM COMPLETE DESCRIPTIONS of your patient's condition. Don't just say, "Sam has glaucoma." Instead, when talking about a specific condition with your team, give detailed descriptions of the symptoms.

● EXPECT A CHANGE IN CLIENTELE. We are in a transition time. People who need a Piscean modality may no longer be comfortable with you and may seek another practitioner. Understand that this might happen and give them a graceful way out. It would be helpful if you put together, for these clients, a list of practitioners who you feel work in the Piscean framework and whom you recommend.

NOTE: Those who are working with teams report that there is a shift in clients but that they end up drawing far more new clients to them. I think there are more people than we realize out there who need this new work and will immediately be drawn to it once they know it is available.

● EXPECT PERSONAL CHANGES as you create and develop this teamwork and the new health system moves along. Use ETS Plus and flower essences to help stabilize yourself and remember to bring any personal issues to your personal MAP team. You won't be eliminating your personal team when you begin working with the professional team. In fact, you may work with your personal team even more. If you are frightened and resistant, and throwing up blocks around the changes that are being suggested in your practice, you can do a MAP/Calibration with your personal team. It's natural for you to have personal responses to the inevitable growing pains and discomfort at working in the dark.

● EXPECT RESISTANCE ON YOUR PART. If you spent years diligently learning a health care system, you will, from time to time, dig your heels in and resist changes your team suggests. This is especially true when the practitioner who opens to the new team has established a reputation. Fear comes up about the possibility of losing recognition or tarnishing a reputation. Also, for a person to work with the MAP team, he has to release a lot of previous knowledge. This, too, can result in a lot of heel digging.

As mentioned above, one excellent way to deal with resistance is to do a MAP/Calibration with your personal team. Do this as soon as you recognize resistance.

*Do not work in a professional team coning while simultaneously having a personal team coning open. Open and work with one coning or the other, not both.*

● THE RIDE OF YOUR LIFE. The impressions shared with me about Professional MAP teams indicates that these teams are excited and anxious to work with us—and they are funny! A number of people have talked about their terrific humor. They are also polite, considerate and caring. However, they will push you a little to keep you moving with the changes.

Perhaps the best thing I've heard many say about Professional MAP is that it is not for the fainthearted. It's amazing to me how often I hear this. People usually get into Professional MAP with the expectation that it will be easy—and immediately are struck by a very different experience. Professional MAP is exciting, exhilarating, demanding, incredibly educational, often amazing, tedious, frustrating, time consuming and sometimes scary. One thing that I think everyone experiencing it would agree on is that it is not easy. The teams are helping you to restructure your health discipline and this will most likely take several years. You will be receiving a huge amount of information, and you will need to test it, work with it, and then integrate it into your practice. There will be times when you will have received so much information that you will need to put the whole thing away and take a breather. This is an *intense* partnership. But many who have stayed with it talk about how liberating this partnership is. You no longer have to know it all. Now you will be working with a team that has the information. You couldn't have a better professional partner than a Professional MAP team.

## ENCOURAGEMENT FROM OTHERS

The following is from a letter I received from an acupuncturist practicing in Ireland. She had been working diligently with her Professional MAP team for about six months when she wrote this. I felt her experiences might be helpful to others.

*. . . Here I'll interject something that may be useful to others —namely, how I ask clients in this conservative area if I can connect to their higher self. After I've done my normal diagnostic work, involving lots of questions and a physical exam, I tell the client that my intent, in all my work, is to work in*

*harmony with that highest part of themselves, however they conceive of it—their spirit, their soul, their higher self. I say that I feel I can do this most effectively if I inwardly ask to consciously connect with them at that level when-ever they are here for a treatment. I ask them if that is alright. When I use this approach, there is unanimous consent—usually with genuine appreciation. I then inwardly do the connecting and disconnecting at each session. This approach has the okay of my Professional MAP team.*

*There are a few clients who I do inform of my work with nature and MAP. Mostly, however, I don't. I think that over time there will be more and more clients I can share with more openly. Naturally, in these cases, I encourage them to work with MAP so as to be able to work on their own as much as they choose and not be dependent on me.*

*Other specific techniques I'm working on with my Professional MAP team include having more than one coning at once. (I have two treatment rooms and sometimes have two clients at the same time—but I don't want the higher self of one to be involved with the other.) I explained to my team what I need, and I have their okay to set up a coning and identify it according to the higher self of the client with whom I'm working. (I just open the initial four-point Professional MAP coning once at the start of the day, and add the client's higher self. Then, if I'm using the second room, I tell my team I need a second treatment room coning* without *John's higher self, and* with *Mary's higher self. If I'm in the room with Mary, and need to get information regarding John (e.g., "Are John's needles ready to come out now?"), I'll ask to switch to John's treatment room coning and then kinesiology test for whatever information I need.*

*Professional MAP teams are not for the fainthearted. It's very difficult to know what's going on when a patient doesn't do well after a treatment. Worst of all, it's hard to rely on my kinesiology testing when I'm asking questions like, "Did I make a mistake in my kinesiology testing for John's treatment?" Usually, I find this is a person I am not supposed to treat. I now try to remember to test for this question before I schedule someone's first appointment. That way, I can refer them to another health professional.*

C.O., Ireland

## PROFESSIONAL MAP SUPPORT

● OUR QUESTION HOT LINE. If you wish to work with a Professional MAP team and have questions about setting it up and getting started with your work with the team, we have a Question Hot Line you can call. We're happy to help you in this most important endeavor. Call our order line or check our web site or catalog for the current Question Hot Line hours.

● PROFESSIONAL MAP NETWORKING LIST. We have established a Professional MAP networking list. If you would like to be on the list and have your contact information made available to other Professional MAP practitioners, just drop us a note letting us know. (This information will not be given to those just working with a personal MAP team.) We suggest that you also let us know what professional discipline you are working in with your team.

If you would like information about other Professional MAP practitioners in your geographic area, let us know this also. We do not automatically send this information when you request to be put on the list.

The Professional MAP networking list is offered so professionals can share with other professionals how they have used MAP in their practices. We ask those requesting it to use it for professional networking only, and not for any advertising or marketing purposes. However, we cannot guarantee that everyone will honor this request.

● SPECIAL CONINGS FOR NON-MEDICAL PROFESSIONS. The Professional MAP procedure described in this chapter is similar to the procedures used for working with nature and a White Brotherhood team in non-medical professions. In these cases, you set up your coning as a "soil-less garden" that specifically applies to the profession you are interested in. We have a complete package of information on how to set up and work in a soil-less garden. *(You do not set up a Professional MAP coning for a non-medical profession.)* For more information on non-medical conings, see Appendix A. For additional soil-less garden information, see our web site or catalog.

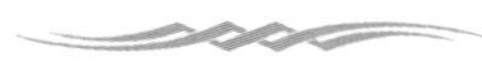

*Chapter 10*

# *Sharing MAP with Others*

IF YOU WISH TO SHARE MAP with others, it is *vital* that you make this entire book available to them and not just the quick-reference MAP steps or your verbal rendition of the steps. It is important that anyone using MAP has the information contained in the book as a foundation. Everyone who gets into the program needs to be fully informed. And they need the information to be unfiltered. This is so they can develop their own relationship with their team in a balanced and safe MAP environment. To give someone just the steps would place them at a serious disadvantage, lead to possible misinterpretation of the steps, and possibly cause them difficulties. MAP is a potent tool and should not be entered into lightly nor should MAP be shared with others in a haphazard manner.

MAP may be the best thing to come along for you. Your life may change in dramatic and exciting ways once you start the work. Because of this, you may have a burning desire to share MAP with everyone you know—and maybe even some you don't know. I ask you to be sensitive about sharing MAP. If you don't know for sure that the other person would be comfortable with the MAP concept and its information, think about it before talking to the person. If you know from past experience that this person will challenge and resist what you would like to say, back off. MAP is a program that is to be embraced heart and soul. It is not a program to sell, convince or do battle over.

## INTRODUCING MAP TO A FRIEND

Besides giving or loaning a friend the book (or suggesting they buy their own copy), you can help by sharing your MAP experiences with this person. And if you are using ETS Plus both as part of MAP and outside the program, talk to your friend about this, as well. Then there's that thoughtful gift idea: Give your friend a copy of *MAP* and a bottle of ETS Plus—and your support.

## INTRODUCING MAP TO AN INFORMAL GROUP

If you wish to present MAP to a group of acquaintances and friends, we ask that you make the book available to the participants at the time of the presentation. Again, it is important that people have access to the full information about MAP and not have to depend on another person's personal interpretation of the program. Sharing the book, your personal experiences and talking about ETS Plus would give them an excellent start to the program. It would also be best if you, as the presenter, have at least six-months experience with your MAP team before presenting MAP to your family and friends. Please call our Perelandra order line for details on making the book available to groups.

## THE MACHAELLE WRIGHT MAP WORKSHOP

I gave an extensive MAP workshop at Perelandra that was taped and is available as a video set. I pulled out the stops about MAP at this workshop because I wanted it to be useful to brand new people as well as those who have worked with MAP for years. It includes:

- How to get started and how to do the program well
- The MAP steps
- Communicating with your team and the art of talking
- Working with MAP in conjunction with other health treatments
- The MAP/Calibration Process
- Kinesiology: how it works, how to use it, helpful hints, pitfalls to avoid and a demonstration of the technique
- Children's MAP
- Professional MAP
- Answers to thirty FAQs about MAP

The video augments the information in this book well.

As I said, this is an extensive workshop. It includes four tapes and I go on for about seven hours. Here's what a lot of people have done with the video. They put together MAP Nights—a series of evenings when a group of interested friends get together, break out the popcorn and chocolate and watch the video, one tape per night. Then they talk about it. With this you have a great support group of friends. Many of these groups continue to meet after viewing the four tapes to talk about their MAP sessions and what they are experiencing.

I think this is a terrific way to get into MAP. This way you begin the program well informed and with a support group. Also, if questions come up during these gatherings that I don't answer in the book or video, we encourage someone from the group to call us during our next Question Hot Line and get the answers to the questions.

## GIVING A MAP WORKSHOP

I don't feel a person is qualified to give a MAP workshop unless they have been working diligently in the program for at least two years. When a person offers a workshop, he implies a certain expertise. I happen to know that there are a number of people who do not meet this criteria and, because they are excited about "spreading the word" or wish to make an easy buck off MAP, feel the need to start a little cottage industry around giving MAP workshops. So, if you think you might like to give a MAP or MAP-related workshop, please meet this two-year-minimum criteria.

The second criteria is that the *MAP* book be made available at the workshop and the participants who are interested in getting into MAP are encouraged to buy the book so that they have the information they need to use the program well. (Contact Perelandra for information about purchasing in quantity.)

The following is an outline for MAP workshops given by two people that is both well put together and maintains MAP's integrity. If you are inclined to offer the program as a workshop, I recommend this format and setup. It has proven to be clear and helpful.

● STEP-BY-STEP OVERVIEW OF THE MAP PROGRAM. In this part each step is given *as written* and discussed. Also include discussions about the White Brotherhood, nature, why both of these groups are involved in a medical program, an explanation of coning, involution/evolution balance, and how the White Brotherhood and nature create involution/evolution balance in the MAP coning.

● TIPS ON WORKING WITH YOUR MAP TEAM. The areas of discussion are taken from Chapter 4 and discussed according to what is written in that chapter and the presenter's personal experiences. Also make sure the participants understand that MAP can be used in conjunction with a doctor's care and how to weave the program in with other trained health care professionals when needed. Make sure they do not feel they must choose one over the other.

● USING KINESIOLOGY TO COMMUNICATE WITH YOUR MAP TEAM. This includes a demonstration of kinesiology and a discussion of the technique and problems they might have with the technique. The information for this is in Appendix B, and expanded on by the presenter's personal experiences with kinesiology. Helping people in a group context to learn kinesiology is easy—after all, it is an easy tool. And it's especially helpful to others because, for some reason, people who do not hesitate for a second to get into MAP will hesitate greatly to learn kinesiology on their own.

● USING ETS PLUS AND FLOWER ESSENCES IN MAP. The basis for this discussion is in Appendix C and also draws from your personal experiences. Our catalog and the video *The Human Electrical System and Flower Essesnces* are also helpful.

### Important Don'ts

- DO NOT OPEN A MAP CONING FOR A GROUP. First of all, this is a misuse of the MAP coning and the teams. MAP is not a group experience. It is a medical program for individuals. Secondly, there are too many unknown variables in a group such as this to assure a safe environment for opening something as powerful as a MAP coning. Someone could panic and experience difficulty. The MAP coning and its members can be discussed in a group context, but the coning itself should not be opened.

- *PLEASE* DO NOT IMPROVISE OR CUSTOMIZE MAP. The MAP program is designed and developed by the White Brotherhood and nature team as it is presented in this book. This is how they wish the program to be used. It is constructed with a strong involution/evolution balance, which is the key to the program's success and ensures optimal safety, efficiency and results. Tinkering with it to suit your personal desires can screw up this balance. If you are presenting the program to others, don't change the MAP steps, the language, or rename any of the team participants. If you are inclined to do these things, you are misrepresenting the program and can cause problems for others.

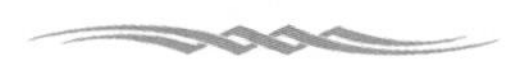

*Chapter 11*

# *Nature Healing Process for Companion Animals*

WHEN IT COMES TO YOUR ANIMALS' health issues, nature is the best and most efficient healing assistant. You can easily set up a healing session for your animal with the Perelandra Nature Healing Process for Companion Animals. Use the Process to address any illness, chronic fear or injury. It may also be used to assist the animal through death. (See Chapter 18 in *The Perelandra Essences* for more information about assisting an animal through its death process.)

NOTE: Use this Process when you know the animal and you choose to participate in its recovery and recuperation. The Process is not set up to be used long distance, therefore you must be physically present with the animal during the session. For helping sick or injured wild animals that are part of your garden's biosphere (should you have a garden), see the "Nature Healing Process for Garden Wildlife" in *The Perelandra Garden Workbook.*

TO PREPARE: You will need a watch or clock with a second hand, pen/pencil and paper for notes, a calendar and ETS for Humans. The full Process will take about an hour (or more, depending on how many questions you ask). You must be physically present with your animal and he or she needs to be quietly lying no closer than three feet from you. Do not hold the animal on your lap or in your hands. This is easy to accomplish if the animal is asleep. However you must remain awake and attentive. You can have a cup of coffee or tea during the Process but eat prior to and not during the session. Also go to the bathroom prior to and not during the session. Don't read, watch TV, play video games or check out your favorite blogs during a session. In short, get comfortable and remain quietly attentive except for those moments when you are directed to say something. When speaking aloud (as directed), you don't have to shout. Just speak loud enough for you to hear yourself.

## THE STEPS

**1A** Set up the Process by stating the following (aloud):
*I would like to set up a Perelandra Nature Healing Process for Companion Animals for ______ (animal's name).*

[Wait five seconds. The Nature Healing Process for Companion Animals team will connect automatically and it is this team you will be working with.]

**1B** To complete the setup, add yourself to the Process by stating (aloud):
*I would like to be included in the Process now.*

[Wait 10 seconds.]

Take one dose (12 drops) of ETS for Humans orally to ensure that you can participate during the Process with strength, clarity and balance.

Your participation in the process is similar to your participation during a vet visit. You will be describing the problem, asking questions, receiving insight and administering any needed post-process assistance.

This completes the setup.

2 Speaking (aloud) to the other members included in the Process setup, describe your animal's condition as fully as possible. Include the circumstances that led to the problem such as a fight, a fall, eating something they should not have, daily separation anxiety, etc. Describe how the animal has reacted. Has it vomited? Has it stopped eating or drinking? Is it listless? Is it favoring a leg? Is it destroying your furniture? Does the animal not wish to be touched or moved? Include all symptoms, changes of normal pattern and reactions that you are observing.

3 Sit quietly with your animal for 40 minutes while the Process team is working. Keep the animal as quiet as possible and maintain a 3-foot distance between the two of you. I repeat: The easiest way to achieve calm and maintain your 3-foot distance is to do the Process while the animal is asleep.

Should any questions or insights come to mind during the 40 minutes, write them down so you won't forget them. Do not ask them during the 40 minutes.

4 After 40 minutes ask your questions and describe any insights you wish to go over. For example, should your animal's diet be changed and how? Is this change temporary? If so, how long should it go on?

One key question you need to always include:

*Will ______ benefit from a vet visit for this situation?*

This is especially important in cases where a bone must be set and stitches or surgery are needed. The point is that there is assistance and technology that vets can easily provide in specific situations. If you get a 'yes' to the above question, it means that for the best care for your companion animal, your Process team wants to work in conjunction with your regular vet.

NOTE: The easiest way to get clean, accurate answers to your questions is by using kinesiology. I recommend you take the time to learn kinesiology so that your participation in the Perelandra Nature Healing Process for Companion Animals will be broader, deeper and more accurate. When you are working with this Process and you don't know how to use kinesiology, still ask the questions and rely on your intuition for answers. Tell your Process team right at the beginning of step 4 and before you ask anything that you will need to get their information intuitively. They will assist your intuition process as much as possible. Doing it this way works, but it leaves more room for misinterpretation. For accuracy, learn to use kinesiology.

Other important questions to ask just before closing down the session in step 5:

*Is an additional Process session needed?*

If yes, ask,

*When is the next session to be scheduled?*

[Point to the days on your calendar, one at a time, and ask, "Is it this day?" Whichever day gets a positive response from kinesiology testing or your intuition is the date for the next session. Be sure to record the day on your calendar.]

**5** Once you've asked all your questions and gone over your insights to make sure you are accurate in your understanding, the session is finished and you will need to deactivate it. Do this by stating (aloud):

*I'd like to close the Perelandra Nature Healing Process for ______ (animal's name) by first removing myself from the Process.*

[Wait 10 seconds.]

Then state (aloud):

*I'd like to complete the deactivation and close down procedure now.*

[Wait 15 seconds.]

Take one dose (12 drops) of ETS for Humans to ensure you are stabilized after participating in this Process session.

The Perelandra Nature Healing Process for Companion Animals is now complete.

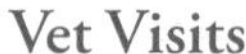

## Vet Visits

As you have probably figured out, it is helpful to include the Perelandra Nature Healing Process team during vet visits. In this situation, the team functions differently than in regular sessions and you do not need to remain three feet away. They will monitor the visit and supply whatever assistance is needed from their perspective as the animal goes through the visit, treatment and any needed boarding stays. To include them, activate only step 1A of the Process just before leaving the house or apartment for the vet appointment. Be sure to let the Process team know you are leaving for the vet appointment. Do not close down the 1A activation until after the animal is back in its home environment. But before closing it down, activate 1B (state "I would like to be added to the Process now.") and ask (aloud):

*Is an additional Process session needed?*

If yes, ask,

*When is the next session to be scheduled?*

[Point to the days on your calendar, one at a time, and ask, "Is it this day?" Whichever day gets a positive response from kinesiology testing or your intuition is the date for the next session. Be sure to record the day on your calendar.]

Repeat these questions at the end of each post-vet session and any regular non-vet session. This will ensure that your animal gets the full benefit from the Process by providing all the sessions it needs for any health issues. When the animal has completely recovered, your answer to the question about additional sessions will be 'no.'

# *Appendices*

*Appendix A*

# Conings

THE KEYSTONE OF MAP IS its coning. It is set up to assure perfect balance between the involution dynamic (nature) and the evolution dynamic (the White Brotherhood and you). The evolution dynamic supplies the definition, direction and purpose to any thing or action. The involution dynamic (nature) supplies the matter, means and action for achieving evolution's definition, direction and purpose. The human soul is the force behind the evolution dynamic. Nature is the force behind involution. In health, the evolution dynamic comes from one's soul. It is from our soul that we receive the impulses that define our direction and our purpose. It is the soul that gives the necessary data to nature for all that is physically required for a human to fully operate within a given lifetime. Nature then supplies our body according to these soul-directed specifications. This also means that nature is the engineer of the human body, and like any good engineer, nature knows how it is supposed to work and how to fix it if it isn't working correctly.

Technically speaking, a coning is a balanced vortex of conscious energy. The simplest way to explain a coning is to say that it is a conference call. With a coning, we are working with more than one intelligence simultaneously.

The reason a coning is needed for multilevel processes is

because of the greater stability, clarity and balance it offers. With multilevel processes, we are working with many different facets and levels of intelligences at one time. Consequently, it is far better to work in an organized team comprised of all those involved in the area we are focusing on.

A coning, by nature, has a high degree of protection built into it. Because of the larger scope of the work, it is important to define exactly who and what are involved in that work. All others are excluded by the mere fact that they have not been activated in the coning. In essence, a coning creates not only the team but also the "room" in which the team is meeting. It is important, when activating a coning, to discern between those team members who are a part of the work to be done and those others who are not involved. The coning is created and activated by us—the human team member. Only those with whom we seek connection will be included. Members will not "slide" in and out of a coning on their own. This adds to the exceptional degree of protection contained within the coning.

I have said that a coning also offers balance and clarity. A friend of mine who began to use a coning whenever she did multilevel work was quite impressed at the difference the coning made in both the quality of her work and the process she went through during her work. She said that when she began to do her work while in a coning, she felt as if she was sitting in a beautiful, sunlit room with the windows open and a lovely warm breeze softly blowing in. Before she learned to use a coning, she would just "connect in" with various "helpers." She said that, in comparison, it was as if she was sitting in a room with no windows and struggling to get a full breath of air. What she was describing was the contrast she felt with the balance and clarity the four-point coning gave her.

Any combination of team members can be activated for the purpose of simultaneous input. But this does not constitute a coning. A true coning has balance built into it. By this I mean a balance between nature and the human soul. In order for us to experience anything fully, we must perceive it in a balanced state; that is, it must have an equal reflection of the soul or spirit dynamics (evolution) combined with an equal reflection of the form/nature dynamics (involution). I see this balance in the shape of a V.

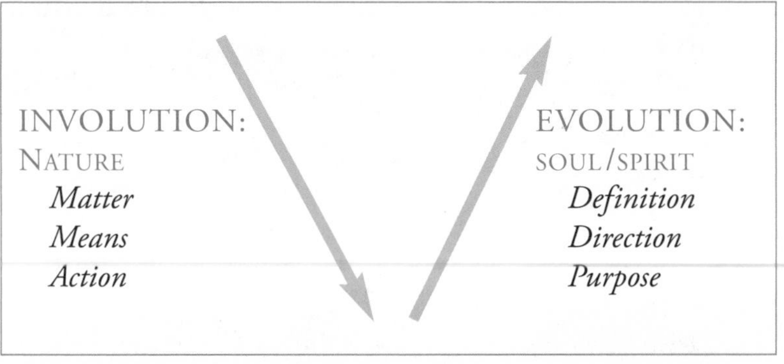


For anything to function well in form, it must have within it a balance between the involution dynamics and the evolution dynamics, or nature and soul. The extent to which we achieve balance between the involution and evolution dynamics depends on our willingness to allow nature to be a partner with us. To have soul and spirit effectively, efficiently and fully activated into form and action, one must have a balance between involution and evolution.

A coning is set up for the purpose of activating a multilevel team for specific work—in this case, MAP. It is therefore important for the successful completion of the work that a balance be maintained between the involution dynamics and the evolution dynamics within the coning itself. We do this by setting up a basic coning, which I call the "four-point coning," that lays a balanced foundation between the involution and evolution dynamics.

As a foundation, the four-point MAP coning maintains the necessary balance between (a) involution/nature, through the connection with the devic and nature spirit levels; and (b) evolution, through the connection with the White Brotherhood Medical Team and the higher self of the person working in the coning. We human souls supply the evolutionary dynamic only. *We cannot supply the involutionary dynamic.*

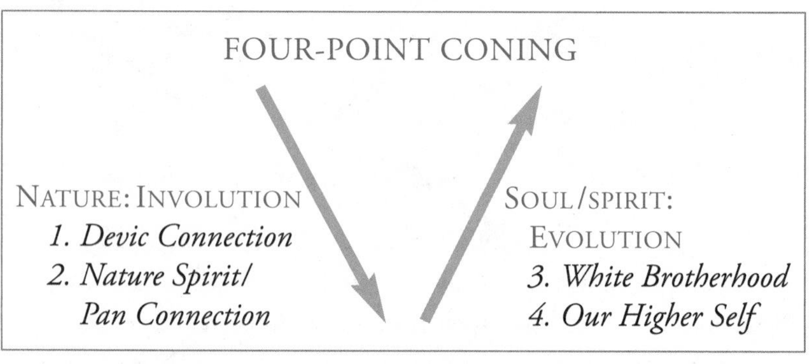


## SOIL-LESS GARDEN CONINGS FOR ALL PROJECTS

A soil-less garden is for those who wish to work with nature and the White Brotherhood in any aspect of their lives: business, education, the arts, the home, research, their job, personal and professional projects and goals... all those gardens in life that are not rooted in soil. A coning may be set up for any project or situation in which we would like good, balanced input and assistance. People also set up conings for assistance in functioning in their occupations. Others set up conings for starting and running their businesses and during all business meetings. With a coning, the meeting runs far more efficiently and decisions are more easily reached. The people who are participating in a coning work with the White Brotherhood to create and hold the appropriate business vision and to define and give purpose to all that needs to be addressed in the meeting. The people then work with nature to come up with solutions and courses of action that best supply the matter, means and action to what they wish to accomplish.

● WHITE BROTHERHOOD. Anyone interested in functioning in harmony with the current transition from the Piscean dynamic to the Aquarian dynamic should include the White Brotherhood in any coning they activate. The White Brotherhood holds the major patterning and rhythms being utilized for this transition. They are part of a balanced coning because they support and assist in ensuring that any work conducted from the coning maintains its forward motion and its connection to the new Aquarian dynamic. For the purpose of a coning other than MAP, it is preferred that we ask, when opening a coning, to be linked with the appropriate members of the White Brotherhood working with __________. (You define the purpose and the area of focus of the coning.) The appropriate members will automatically be activated in the coning. If you aren't clear about what or who to ask for, just ask for a *general connection to the White Brotherhood.* This will create a general, nonspecific connection with them that will ensure that the evolutionary dynamic in the coning is consistent with the intent and direction of the new Aquarian shift.

- HIGHER SELF. In all conings, we include our higher self to assure that the work done is compatible with our higher direction and purpose. This input is given automatically by the fact that our higher self is linked into the coning.

- DEVIC. The devic connection of the coning ensures that the work being done maintains an overall integrity with nature's design in the area in which we are working. The devic level also creates or designs appropriate courses of action and solutions to specific situations or problems that need addressing. Each coning has in it a specific deva. For example, the MAP coning has the Overlighting Deva of Healing. NOTE: A deva is "overlighting" if it is the "chief" deva of a larger devic team. Each area of healing has its own deva. The deva that "coordinates and oversees" all these areas is the overlighting deva. But you don't have to get bogged down with semantics. If you wish to work with the deva of your business, or the deva of your home, just ask for the deva of __________. You don't have to know if it's overlighting or not. When opening a coning, think about what issue or situation you wish to address in the coning, then ask to be connected with the deva of that specific issue or situation.

For some situations, you may need more than one deva. A four-point coning only refers to the divisions of the coning. It does not mean only four members can participate in a coning. In some cases, you may need to identify situations within larger contexts, and include several devas as a result. For example, if I wish to work in a coning with a specific vegetable in the Perelandra garden, I will include the Deva of Perelandra, the Deva of the Perelandra Garden and the deva of the specific vegetable in question. These three devas constitute one point of the coning. And, the fact that I have three devas "standing on that point," doesn't overload the point or give it additional "weight." Another example: Several years ago, one of my staff put together a team training program for us. To do this, she worked in a four-point coning. For the devic point, she included the Deva of Perelandra (to maintain the overall direction and intent of Perelandra), the Deva of the Perelandra Business (representing the business direction and intent) and the Deva of Team Development. These three devas combined to create the appropriate team-development program for the Perelandra business staff.

● PAN. The nature spirit point of the coning is connected through Pan. We do this because all nature spirit levels except Pan are regional, and rather than try to figure out which nature spirit levels are involved in the work we wish to do, we work with Pan—the one nature spirit level that is universal in dynamic and is involved in all of the nature spirit activities. Pan's connection helps us maintain integrity with natural law for all action and issues worked on in the coning and gives assurance that the nature spirit activity and input is fully represented at all times.

I'm giving you the steps for opening a four-point coning for yourself. But I strongly recommend that before you launch into working in a coning with your business, job, home, art, classes, etc., you have more information than I am able to give you here. I have given a workshop on soil-less gardens and I highly recommend you get the video of this workshop: *Working with Nature in Soil-less Gardens.* (See our web site or catalog for more information on soil-less gardens and this video.)

The workshop includes:

- Why it is important to work with nature in soil-less gardens
- Our conscious partnership with nature, how it works and why it works
- Our role and nature's role in the partnership
- How the two roles operate together
- What a coning is, how to "construct" a balanced coning for a soil-less garden and work with it
- How to initiate and activate a soil-less garden
- How to work with nature to achieve your goal
- Pitfalls to watch out for
- Using kinesiology with the coning: how it works, how to do kinesiology and several testing demonstrations.

## OPENING A FOUR-POINT CONING

Have your bottle of ETS Plus handy.

1 State: *I would like to open a coning.*

2 Link with each appropriate member of the coning individually. Wait ten seconds after each connection.

- The specific deva(s) involved
- Pan
- The White Brotherhood—State: *I'd like to be connected with the appropriate members of the White Brotherhood working with* __________ .*

- Your higher self—State: *I'd like my higher self to be connected to the coning.*

Wait another ten to fifteen seconds after activating the full coning so that your body can stabilize itself within the coning and with the team.

*For a non-medical professional White Brotherhood coning (as described in Chapter 9), state that you wish to shift your work to include the new Aquarian dynamic and want to work in a professional White Brotherhood team to accomplish this. Then describe your professional area.

3 Take one dose of ETS Plus to make sure that the process of activating a coning did not affect your balance.

4 Do the work or have the meeting you desire.

5 When the work is completed, thank your team for its assistance, and close down or dismantle the coning. *Closing down is important.* You do this simply by stating you would like to be disconnected from:

- Your higher self
- The White Brotherhood
- Pan
- The specific deva(s) involved

6 Take another dose of ETS Plus, just to be sure that you held your balance once the coning work was completed.

A four-point coning closes automatically as soon as you request the disconnections. No member is going to resist a disconnection any more than they would resist a connection. You are the one in command of the creation, activation and dismantling of the coning.

## IMPORTANT POINTS ABOUT CONINGS

● MULTIPLE MEMBERS. You may include as many members in your team as you like and maintain involution/evolution balance as long as you begin with the regular four-point coning as your foundation. However, it is best to include only those who are directly related to the work being done. Some people get a little crazy about coning activation and add forty-two members who might possibly be involved or might like to be involved. If you do, you no longer have a tight, cohesive team. You now have a mob coning instead.

I urge you to resist activating a mob coning for two reasons:

- It is totally unnecessary and does not strengthen or enhance a coning in any way.
- *You,* as the initiator and activator of the coning, will feel a substantial physical drain as you try to hold a coning with an unnecessary number of members present throughout the time it takes for the process or work.

A coning, although invisible, is a physical energy reality that will interact with you. A mob coning would require the same amount of energy as trying to hold a deep conversation with six people in the middle of the New York Stock Exchange on Friday afternoon. You are going to feel exhausted from this kind of overload. So, the key to "good coning building" is to be precise about who you request to be on the team. Each member should have an integral role in the work to be done.

There's another point. *No other person's higher self should be added into a coning without his or her conscious permission.* To do so without conscious permission from that person is just plain rude and ethically wrong.

Because working in a coning is a physical phenomenon for us, we need to address some basic physical needs.

● CONING HOURS. Normally, we should not work in a coning for more than *one hour at a time.* This is especially true in the beginning when we are getting used to working with and in a coning. Your body needs time to adjust to this new dynamic. If you need to do more than can be accomplished within the one-hour time frame, close down the coning and continue in a new coning later that day or the next day.

● PROTEIN DRAIN. Activating, working with and dismantling a coning require sharp focus on our part. As a result, we may experience a protein drain. You will know you are experiencing such a drain if you come out of the coning and are suddenly attacked with a galloping case of the munchies. Often, we translate a protein drain into a desire for sweets. I have nothing against a great big piece of chocolate from time to time. But in this case, you need protein to compensate for the drain. Then eat your chocolate.

HINT: Have a bag of nuts with you while you are in a coning and occasionally down a few. This will avoid or minimize the protein drain while you are in the coning.

Also, I find that while in the coning, I do not perceive the protein drain or any hunger. It doesn't register until after I close down the coning. So I suggest that, if you are not hungry during the coning, don't let that fool you. Still have your supply of nuts handy, and eat a few throughout the session.

- TAKING BREAKS WHILE IN AN OPEN CONING. If you need to take a break during a coning session, do not close the coning and then re-open it. Just tell your team that you need a break for fifteen minutes or a half-hour or whatever (don't make it a vacation). They will automatically shift the coning into what I call the "at-rest" position. You may feel the intensity of the coning back off a bit when this shift occurs. It will take about five seconds. Then have your break. When you are ready to resume, announce that your break is over and that you would like to fully activate the coning again, and the coning will automatically shift back into its previous active connection and intensity.

- JUNK CONING SESSIONS. Don't get into the habit of activating conings indiscriminately. They are to be used for inter-level work, and not for prediction-type information. Your coning members are functioning in a team dynamic with you and do not wish to be asked to function in areas where your common sense should be the dominant factor. Opening a coning to ask if you should go on a specific vacation or if it would be good for you to invest money in a certain stock is not appropriate. As far as your team is concerned, such decisions are best left to your common sense and intelligence.

- KEEPING IT CURRENT. I also suggest that you limit the questions to issues that pertain to the present. Information about the future is reliable only if *all* issues and elements involved remain *exactly* the same as they were when you asked your questions. In a changing world populated by six billion people with active free wills, this never happens. By the time you get to some future point in time, all issues and elements will most likely have changed perspective and position. Therefore your answers about what to do will also need to change. In short, it is a waste of time and a crapshoot to try to see into the future—from within a coning or otherwise.

● NO CONING NEEDED. There is something else I would like to explain. Many people use kinesiology to discern issues about themselves. For example, they may wish to know if they are to take a certain vitamin. This is a question that can be accurately answered using kinesiology and should not be addressed in a soil-less garden coning. If you want to know whether you should wear yellow or red for a special occasion in order to enhance your strength and balance, *your* electrical system has the answer. Either your electrical system is strong when you hold that color or it is weak. A simple kinesiology test will accurately discern this for you. You don't need to call a team meeting.

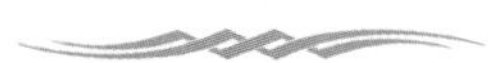

*Appendix B*

# *Kinesiology: The Tool for Testing*

KINESIOLOGY IS ANOTHER NAME for muscle testing. And it is simple. Anybody can do it because it uses your electrical system and your muscles. If you are alive, you have these two things. I know that sounds smart-mouthed of me, but I've learned that sometimes people refuse to believe that anything can be so simple. So they create a mental block—only "sensitive types" can do this, or only women can do this. It's not true. Kinesiology happens to be one of those simple things in life just waiting around to be learned and used by everyone.

I don't mean to intimidate you, but small children can learn to do kinesiology in about five minutes. It's mainly because it never occurred to them that they couldn't do it. If I tell them they have an electrical system, they don't argue with me about it—they just get on with the business of learning how to do simple testing. Actually, I *do* mean to intimidate you. Your first big hurdle will be whether or not you believe you have a viable electrical system that is capable of being tested. Here's a good test: Place a hand mirror under your nose. If you see breath marks, you have a strong electrical system. (If you don't see breath marks, call 911—you're in trouble.) Now you can get on with learning how to use kinesiology.

If you've ever been to a chiropractor or holistic physician experienced in muscle testing, you've experienced kinesiology. The doctor tells you to stick out your arm and resist his pressure. It feels as if he is trying to push your arm down after he has told you not to let him do it. Everything is going fine, and then all of a sudden he presses and your arm flops down like an old fish. He is using kinesiology.

Simply stated, the body has within it and surrounding it an electrical network or grid. If a negative energy (that is, any physical object or energy that does not maintain or enhance health and balance) is introduced into a person's energy field, his muscles, when having physical pressure applied, are unable to hold their strength. (The ability to hold muscle power is directly linked to the balance of the electrical system.) In other words, if pressure is applied to an individual's extended arm while his field is affected by a negative (energy), the arm will not be able to resist the pressure. It will weaken and fall to his side. If pressure is applied while affected by a positive (energy), the person will easily resist the pressure and the arm will hold its position.

When a negative is placed in a person's energy field, his electrical system will immediately respond by short-circuiting or overloading. This makes it difficult for the muscles to maintain their strength and hold the position when any pressure is added. When a positive is placed within a person's energy field, the electrical system holds, and the muscles maintain their strength when pressure is applied.

This electrical/muscular relationship is a natural part of the human system. It is not mystical or magical. And for many practitioners, kinesiology is the established method for reading that balance.

If you have ever experienced muscle testing, you most likely participated in the above-described, two-person operation. You provided the extended arm, and the other person provided the pressure. Although efficient, this can be cumbersome when you want to test something on your own. Arm pumpers have the habit of disappearing when you need them. So you will be learning to self-test—no arm pumpers needed.

## SELF-TESTING STEPS

1 THE CIRCUIT FINGERS. If you are right-handed: Place your left hand palm up. Connect the tip of your left thumb with the tip of the left little finger. (Not your index finger. I'm talking about your thumb and little finger.) If you are left-handed: Place your right hand palm up. Connect the tip of your right thumb with the tip of your right little finger. By connecting your thumb and little finger, you have just closed a major electrical circuit in your hand, and it is this circuit you will use for testing.

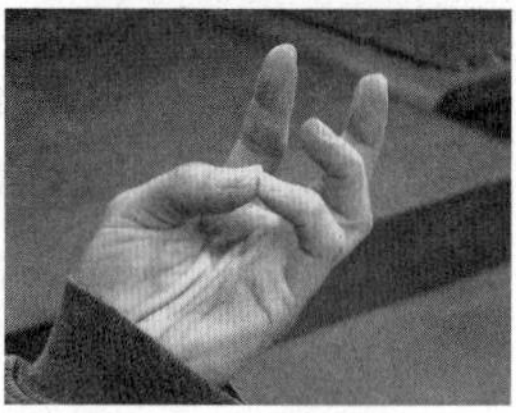

Before going on, look at the position you have just formed with your hand. If your thumb is touching the tip of your index or finger #1, laugh at yourself for not being able to follow directions and change the position so you touch the tip of the

*Fig. 1: Circuit fingers–tip to tip*

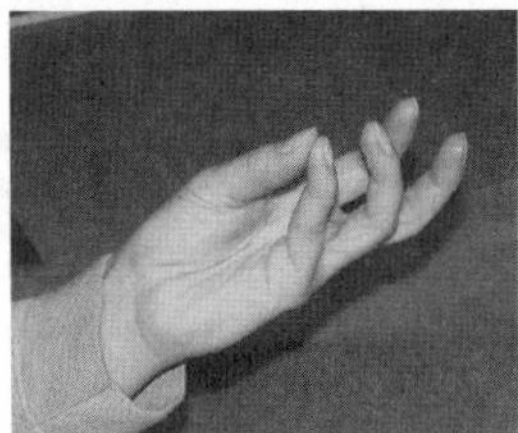

Fig. 2: Circuit fingers–pad to pad

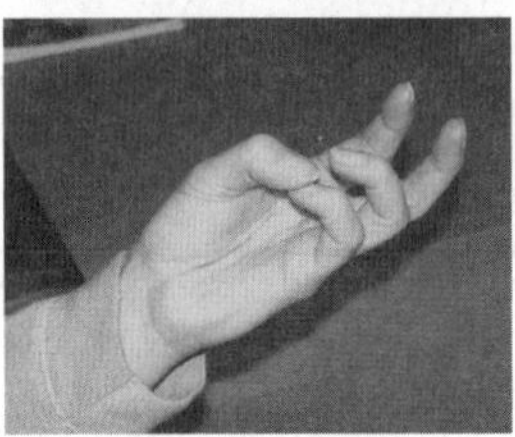

Fig. 3: Circuit fingers–thumb over little finger

thumb with the tip of the little finger. Most likely this will not feel at all comfortable to you. This is because you normally don't put your fingers in this position and they might feel a little stiff. If you are feeling awkwardness, you've got the first step of the test position! In time, the hand and fingers will adjust to being put in this position and it will feel fine.

Circuit fingers can touch tip to tip *(Fig. 1)*, finger pad to pad *(Fig. 2)*, or thumb resting on top of the little finger's nail *(Fig. 3)*. I rest my thumb on top of my little finger. And I suggest this position for anyone with long nails. You're not required to impale yourselves for this.

When you have the circuit fingers in the correct position, they form a circle. If you straighten fingers 1, 2 and 3 a bit, you will get them out of the way and you will see the circle.

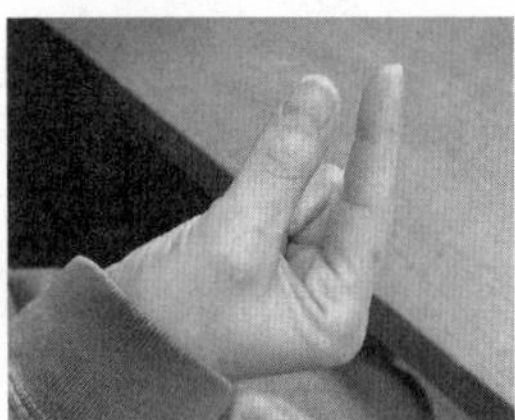

Fig. 4: The test fingers

2 THE TEST FINGERS AND TESTING POSITION. To test the circuit (the means by which you will apply pressure), place the test fingers, thumb and index finger of your other hand *(Fig. 4)*, *inside* the circle you have created by connecting your circuit thumb and little finger. The test fingers (thumb/index fingers) should be right under the circuit fingers (thumb/little fingers), touching them, with your test thumb resting against the underside of your circuit thumb and your test index finger resting against the underside of your circuit little finger. *(Fig. 5)*

Don't try to make a circle with your test fingers. They are just placed inside the circuit fingers that do form a circle. It will look like you have two "sticks" inserted inside a circle.

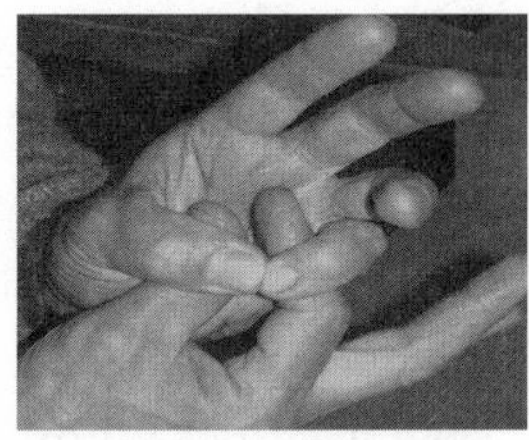

*Fig. 5: The testing position*

3 Positive response. Keeping this position, ask yourself a simple question in which you already know the answer to be "yes." ("Is my name _____?") Once you've asked the question, press your circuit fingers together, keeping them in the circular position. *Using the same amount of pressure,* try to press apart or separate the circuit fingers with your test fingers. Press the lower thumb against the upper thumb, and the lower index finger against the upper little finger. (The action of your test fingers will look like scissors separating as you apply pressure to your circuit fingers. Your testing fingers, the fingers inserted in the circuit circle, will remain in position within the circle. *(Figs. 6 and 7)* All you are doing is using these two testing fingers to apply pressure to the outer two circuit fingers. Don't try to pull your test fingers vertically up through your circuit fingers.)

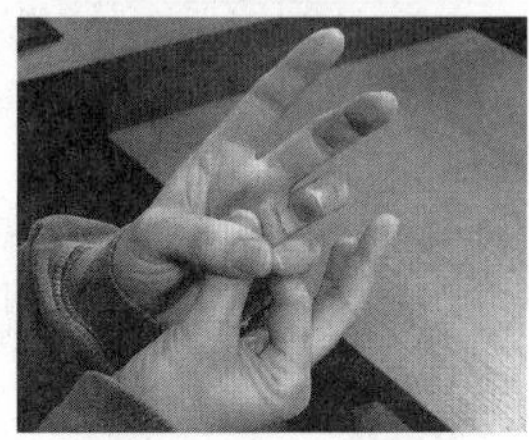

*Fig. 6: Positive response with the circuit fingers still closed*

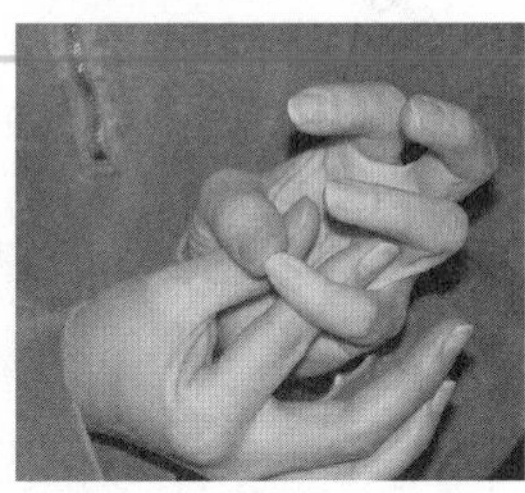

*Fig. 7: Another view of the positive response*

The circuit position described in step 1 corresponds to the position you take when you stick your arm out for the physician. The testing position in step 2 is in place of the physician or other convenient arm pumper. After you ask the yes/no question and you press your circuit fingers tip-to-tip, that is equal to the doctor saying, "Resist my pressure." Your circuit fingers now correspond to your outstretched, stiffened arm. Trying to push apart those fingers with your testing fingers is equal to the doctor pressing down on your arm.

If the answer to the question is positive (if your name is what you think it is!), you will not be able to easily push apart the circuit fingers. The electrical circuit will hold, your muscles will maintain their strength and your circuit fingers will not separate. You will feel the strength in that circuit.

● Calibrating the finger pressure. The amount of pressure holding the circuit fingers together must be *equal* to the amount of your testing fingers pressing against them. Also, do not use a pumping action (pressing against your circuit fingers several times in rapid succession) when applying pressure to your circuit fingers. Use an equal and continuous pressure.

Play with this a bit. Ask a few more yes/no questions that have positive answers. Now, I know it is going to seem that if you already know the answer to be "yes," you are probably "throwing" the test. Well, you are. This is your tool for calibrating your fingers for feeling the strong positive. You are asking yourself a question that has a positive answer. If your circuit fingers are separating, you are applying too much pressure with your testing fingers. Or you are not putting enough pressure into holding your circuit fingers together. You need to keep asking the question and play with the testing until you feel pressure in all four fingers and the pressure in your testing fingers is not separating your circuit fingers. You don't have to break or strain your fingers for this; just use enough pressure to make them feel alive, connected and alert. When this happens, now you have a clear positive kinesiology response.

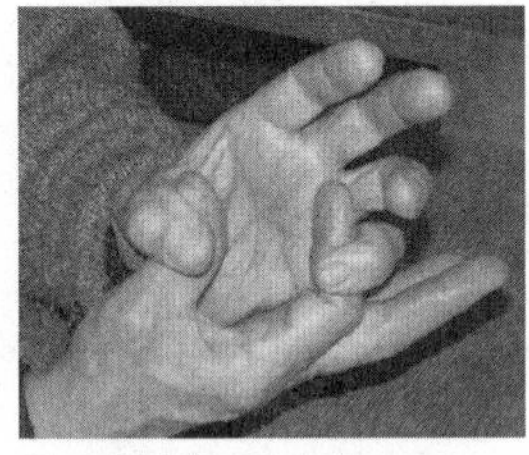

*Fig. 8: Negative response–a lot of separation*

4 NEGATIVE RESPONSE. Once you have a clear sense of the positive response, ask yourself a question that has a negative answer. Again press your circuit fingers together and now, using equal pressure, press against the circuit fingers with the test fingers. This time, if the testing-fingers' pressure is equal to the circuit-fingers' pressure, the electrical circuit will break and the circuit fingers will weaken and separate. Because the electrical circuit is broken, the muscles in the circuit fingers do not have the power to hold the fingers together. In a positive state the electrical circuit holds, and the muscles have the power to keep the two fingers together.

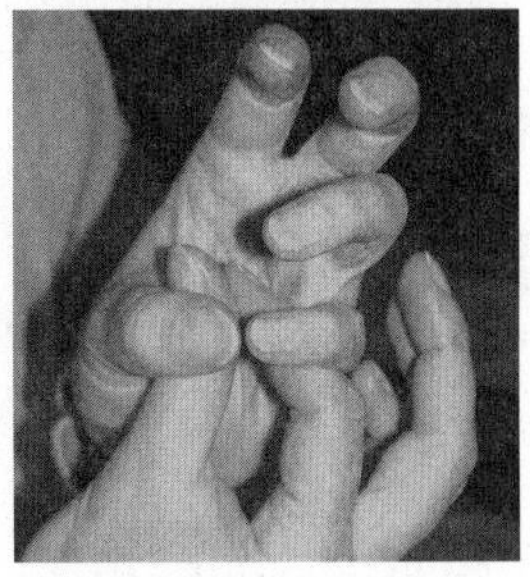

*Fig. 9: Negative response–a little separation*

● DIFFERENT STYLES IN HOW THE FINGERS SEPARATE.

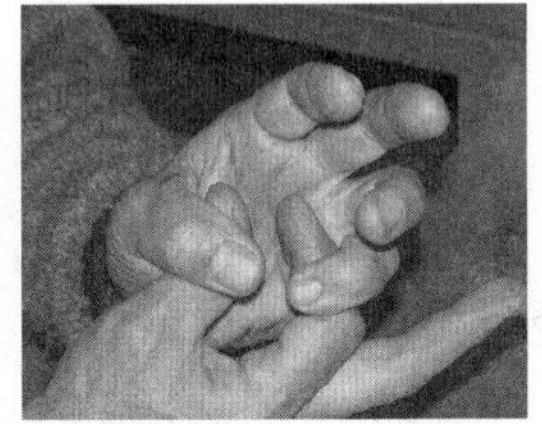

*Fig. 10: Negative response–medium separation*

How much your circuit fingers separate depends on your personal style. Some people's fingers separate a lot. *(Fig. 8)* Other's barely separate at all. (Fig. 9) Mine separate about a quarter of an inch. *(Fig. 10)* Some people's fingers won't separate at all, but they'll definitely feel the fingers weaken when pressure is applied during a "no" answer. Let your personal style develop.

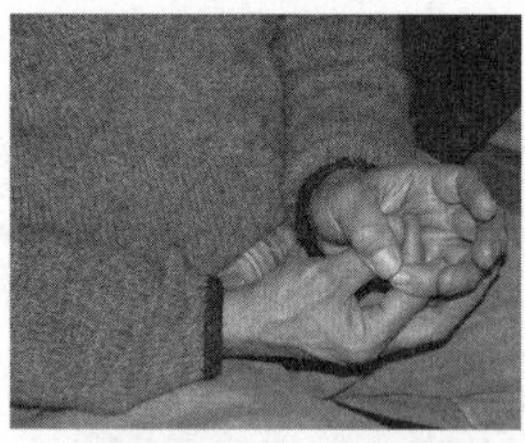
*Fig. 11: Forearms resting in a person's lap while testing*

● RESTING YOUR FOREARMS. If you are having a little trouble feeling anything, do your testing with your forearms resting in your lap. *(Fig. 11)* This way you won't be using your muscles to hold your arms up while you are trying to test.

● CALIBRATING THE NEGATIVE RESPONSE. To calibrate and equalize the pressure used by the circuit fingers and the testing fingers for negative responses, play with negative questions and continue adjusting the pressure between your circuit and test fingers until you get a clear negative response.

When you're feeling a solid separation, return to positive questions. Once again, get a good feeling for the strength between your circuit fingers when the electricity is in a positive state. Then ask a negative question and feel the weakness when the electricity is in a negative state. Practice your testing by alternating the questions.

In the beginning, you may feel only a slight difference between the two. With practice, that difference will become more pronounced. For now, it is just a matter of trusting what you have learned—and practicing.

● THE TESTING CALIBRATION. Especially in the beginning, and even sometimes after you have been doing kinesiology successfully for awhile, you may lose the strong feeling of the positive response and the weakness of the negative. You've lost the equal pressure between your circuit and testing fingers and one set is overpowering the other.

When this happens, just back away from whatever you are trying to test and do a testing calibration. Ask yourself a question that you know has a positive answer and test for the response. Adjust the pressure between your testing and circuit fingers until you feel a strong, positive response. Play with this a bit and get a feel for the strength of the positive responses.

Then switch to questions that have a negative response and play around with the pressure until you feel a clear breaking of the circuit.

After this, alternate your questions between positive and negative a few times and test the answer. In no time, you'll have the "kinesiology feel" back and you can resume testing where you left off. (See p. 244, "Calibrating Your Fingers.")

Don't forget the overall concept behind kinesiology. What enhances our body, mind and soul makes us strong. Together, our body, mind and soul create a holistic environment that, when balanced, is strong and solid. If something enters that environment and negates or challenges the balance, the environment is weakened. That strength or weakness registers in the electrical system, and it can be discerned through a muscle-testing technique—kinesiology.

## KINESIOLOGY TIPS

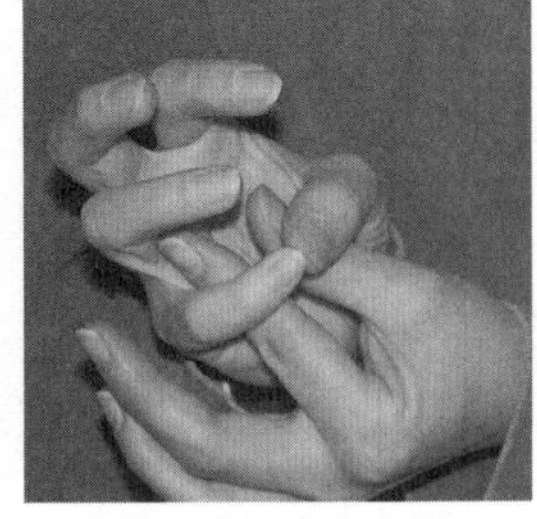

*Opposite hands with circuit fingers–tip to tip*

THE NEED TO SWITCH HANDS. If you are having trouble feeling the electrical circuit in the circuit fingers, try switching hands —the circuit fingers become the test fingers and vice versa. Most people who are right-handed have this particular electrical circuitry in their left hand. Left-handers generally have the circuitry in their right hand. But sometimes a right-hander has the circuitry in the right hand and a left-hander has it in the left hand. Or some heavy-handed teacher along the way forbid you to write with the left hand and required you to learn to write with your right hand. You may be one of those people. If you are ambidextrous, choose the circuit hand that gives you the clearest responses. Before deciding which to use, give yourself a couple of weeks of testing using one hand as the circuit hand to get a good feel for its responses before trying the other hand.

● KINESIOLOGY TESTING AND INJURIES. If you have an injury such as a muscle sprain in either hand or arm, don't do kinesiology testing until you have healed. Kinesiology is muscle testing, and a muscle injury will interfere with the testing—and the testing will interfere with the healing of the muscle injury.

## An Alternative Kinesiology Testing Method

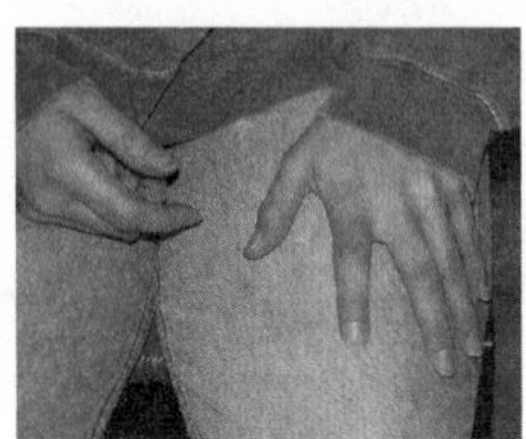

*Fig. 12: Connecting the finger-to-thigh circuits*

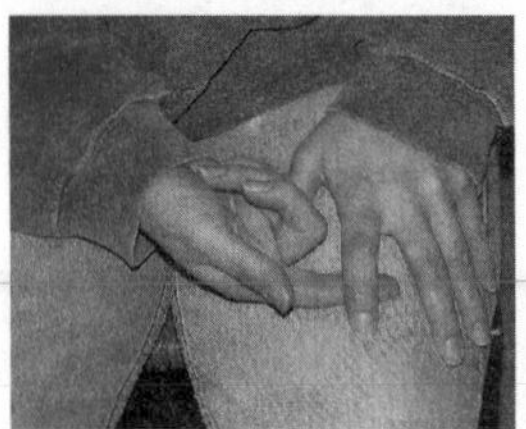

*Fig. 13: The alternative testing position*

There is a method of kinesiology that uses the pointing finger of your test hand and your leg. If you have a physical impairment, this may be easier for you to use.

1 CONNECTING THE CIRCUIT. Place the pointing finger (index finger) of your test hand on top of the center of your thigh. (Left test hand rests on left thigh or right test hand on right thigh.) This finger should lay flat on the leg. Your other fingers may be in whatever position is comfortable. *(Fig. 12)*

2 THE TESTING POSITION. Place the pointing finger of the other hand in a face-up position under the first knuckle of the test finger. *(Fig. 13)* Make sure you are using the knuckle section, not just the tip of the finger (the first knuckle of these two fingers should be in contact).

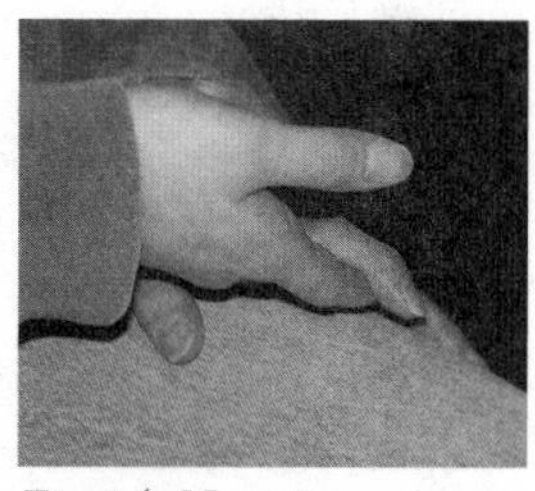

*Fig. 14: Negative response –the test finger lifts*

The circuit that you're using runs down the center of the leg and you are connecting it with the circuit in your finger.

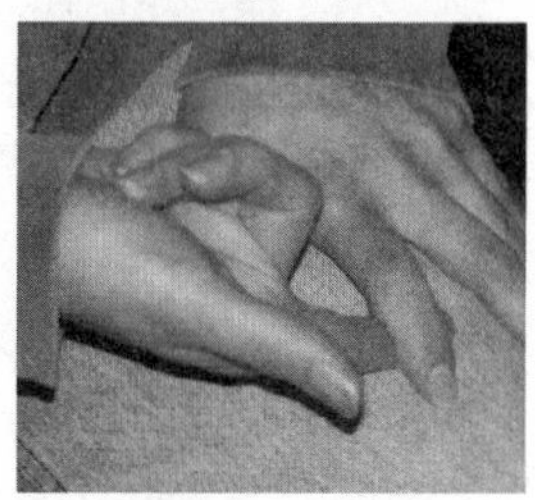

*Fig. 15: Positive response –the test finger remains connected*

3 TO TEST. Ask the question, press your test finger down on the leg, then, using equal pressure, try to lift up the finger of the test hand.

If the circuit breaks easily and the testing finger lifts, the answer is negative. *(Fig. 14)* If the circuit holds and it is difficult to lift the test finger, the answer is positive. *(Fig. 15)*

● LEARNING KINESIOLOGY IN THE RIGHT ENVIRONMENT. When first learning kinesiology, do yourself a favor and set aside some quiet time to go through the instructions and play with the testing. Trying to learn this while riding the New York subway during evening rush hour isn't going to give you the break you need. But once you have learned it, you will be able to test all kinds of things while riding the subway.

● THE KINESIOLOGY BODY/MIND CONNECTION. Sometimes I meet people who are trying to learn kinesiology and are not having much luck. They've gotten frustrated, decided this isn't for them and have gone on to try to learn another means of testing. Well, I'll listen to them explain what they did, and before they know it, I've verbally tricked them with a couple of suggestions about their testing, which they try, and they begin feeling kinesiology for the first time—a strong "yes" and a clear "no." The problem wasn't kinesiology. Everyone, as I have said, has an electrical system. The problem was that they wanted to learn it so much that they became overly anxious and tense—and they blocked.

Since you won't have me around to trick you, if you suspect you're blocking, go on to something else. Then trick yourself. You'll need to get your head out of the way. When you care the least about whether or not you learn kinesiology, start playing with it again. Approach it as if it were a game. That's when you'll feel the strength and weakness in the fingers.

## Troubleshooting Your Testing

Suppose the testing has been working fine, and then suddenly you can't get a clear result (what I call a "definite maybe") or you get no result at all. Check the following:

- SLOPPY TESTING. You try to press apart the fingers *before* applying pressure between the circuit fingers. This happens especially when we've been testing for awhile and become overconfident or do the testing very quickly. I think it happens to all of us from time to time and serves to remind us to keep our attention on the matter at hand. (Excuse the pun.)

Especially in the beginning, start a kinesiology session by first feeling a few positive and negative responses. Ask yourself some of those obvious questions. Or simply say several times,

"Let me feel a positive." (Test.) "Let me feel a negative." (Test.) This will serve as a kind of warm-up and remind you what positive and negative feel like before you start. If the testing begins to feel sloppy in the middle of some work, stop the testing and do a kinesiology calibration to get the pressure equalized on both hands again. (See p. 244.)

● EXTERNAL DISTRACTIONS. Trying to test in a noisy or active area can cause you to lose concentration. The testing will feel unsure or contradict itself if you double-check the results. Often, moving to a quiet, calm spot and concentrating on what you are doing will be just what's needed for successful testing.

● FOCUS OR CONCENTRATION. Even in a quiet spot, one's mind may wander and the testing will feel fuzzy, weak or contradictory. It is important to concentrate throughout the process. Check how you are feeling. If you're tired, I suggest you not try to test until you have rested a bit. And if you have to go to the bathroom, do it. That situation is a sure concentration-destroyer.

● THE QUESTION ISN'T CLEAR. A key to kinesiology is asking a simple yes/no question, not two questions in one, each having a possible yes/no answer. If your testing isn't working, first check your hand positions. Next, review your question, and make sure you are asking only one question. And, while you're asking a question, don't think ahead to the next question! Your fingers won't know which to answer.

● MATCH YOUR INTENT WITH YOUR WORDING. If you are prone to saying, "Oh, I didn't mean to say that!" when you talk to others, this might be an area you need to work on.

A woman at one of our workshops asked me about some strange answers she had gotten about what to feed her cat. She had asked, "What kinds of food would make my cat happy?" She got weird answers like chocolate, catnip, sirloin steak... I pointed out that she probably asked the wrong question. She meant to ask what foods would make her cat healthy. She was a little surprised. She thought that this was the question she had originally asked. In short, her question and her intent did not match.

- YOU MUST WANT TO ACCEPT THE RESULTS. If you enter a kinesiology test not wanting to "hear" the answer, for whatever reason, you can override the test with your emotions and your will. This is true for conventional situations as well. If you don't want something to work for you, it won't work. That's our personal power dictating the outcome.

- TESTING EMOTIONAL MINEFIELDS. If you are trying to do testing during a situation that is especially emotional for you, that deeply stirs your emotions, or if you are trying to ask a question in which you have a strong, personal investment in the answer—such as, "Should I buy this beautiful $850,000 house?"—I suggest that you not test until you are calmer or get some emotional distance from the situation. During such times, you are walking a very fine line between a clear test and a test that your desires are overriding. Kinesiology as a tool is not the issue here. It is the condition or intent of the tester. In fact, some questions just shouldn't be asked, but which questions shouldn't be asked is relative to who is doing the asking. We each need to develop discernment around which questions are appropriate for us to ask.

When I am involved with testing during emotionally stressful times, I stop for a moment, collect my thoughts and make a commitment to concentrate on the testing only. And if I must test an emotionally charged question or a question about something I have a personal investment in, I stop a moment, commit myself to the test—and to receiving the answer and not the answer I might desire.

IMPORTANT: I suggest that you make it a rule not to ask questions like "Do I have cancer?" Your ability to perceive the answer either through kinesiology or intuition is questionable. It is too emotionally charged. If you have a suspicion, get a solid diagnosis from the allopathic medical establishment, and make sure you get two or three "second opinions."

● A SUDDEN BREAKDOWN OF YOUR TESTING. If your testing has been going along just fine and you suddenly begin to get contradictory or "mushy" test results, consider that this may not be a good day for you to do this particular work.

- You could be too tired to hold your focus on the testing.
- Or you may need to drink water! If you are dehydrated, your electrical system will feel weak during kinesiology testing. You just need to put water in your battery.
- Or you may need to test yourself for flower essences. The essences balance and repair the electrical system, and this may be just what you need for clear kinesiology results.

● ODD RESULTS. If your testing results seem odd (you're getting all negative responses or all positive responses), you need to back away from the testing and take a short break. You are nervous, distracted, in need of water and/or tired.

- If you are tired, take a short break, eat some protein and return to the testing where you left off or start the testing again from the top if you're not sure about the accuracy of your previous testing.
- If you are distracted, take a short break, do what you need to do to eliminate the distraction and return to the testing where you left off.
- If you are nervous, take a short break, regroup, give yourself a pep talk and relax. If you need water, drink. Then return to the testing where you left off.

## Calibrating Your Fingers

Before resuming the testing, "calibrate your fingers" and get the feel for your kinesiology yes/no responses.

1 Do this by first asking yourself a question you already know the answer to and is guaranteed to give you a positive response, such as "Is my name _________?" Now test.

2 If you don't get the positive response, your fingers need calibrating. The pressure you are using on both hands isn't equal.

3 Adjust the pressure (back off the pressure you are exerting to hold the circuit fingers together or the pressure you're exerting with the two testing fingers) until you get a clear, strong positive response.

4 Then ask the question and continue adjusting the pressure when needed.

5 Do this until you feel you're getting a consistent positive response to your question.

6 Now repeat this process, only this time ask a question that you know will give you a negative response. "Do I weigh 1863 pounds?" Or "Is my name Donald Duck?" (If your name is actually Donald Duck, you'll need to pick another false name, like "Minnie Mouse.") Continue with the kinesiology calibration process until you feel you're getting a consistent negative response to your question. Then resume the testing.

● SEQUENTIAL TESTING. You use sequential kinesiology testing when you need to find out how many times you should do something, how many days you should do something, how many drops of something you need... information that suggests a pattern. To get this information, you need to set up your kinesiology testing a little differently. Let's say you are working with Professional MAP and you need to find out how many more monitoring sessions your team is requesting. Address the question to your coning and set up the testing like this:

*Do you want one more monitoring session?* (Test.)

If yes, ask,

*Do you want two more monitoring sessions?* (Test.)

If yes, ask,

*Three more?* (Test.)

Do a count until you get a negative response. Let's say your team wants three monitoring sessions. You tested positive for one, then two and then three. When you tested for four, you got a negative response. This means the correct answer was three. The team wants three sessions and not four.

● How your MAP team uses kinesiology to communicate with you. This is simple. Whenever you want information from your team, pose it in a simple yes/no question. If the answer is yes, the team will project a positive energy into your electrical system. When you test that question, your circuits will remain strong and you will receive a positive result. If the answer is no, they will project the negative energy of "no" into your system, your circuits will weaken and you will receive a negative result. To get more complex information from your team using kinesiology, you will need to ask a series of questions. This is when it is especially important to keep notes of the questions and answers you get. Once you try asking a series of questions a few times, you'll see how much information you can get directly from your MAP team and will want to have these kinesiology Q&A times with them more often. With a little practice, the kinesiology Q&A sessions will smooth out and your ability to ask good questions and test the answers quickly will improve. Many people using this method feel like they are having a "normal" conversation with their team and that kinesiology is not a hindrance at all. It just takes practice and patience.

● If you are having trouble learning kinesiology. Ask your MAP team for help. Explain what's happening and your frustrations around learning the technique. And finally, we're not of the same caliber as a MAP team, but we'll be happy to help you out also. Just call our Question Hot Line.

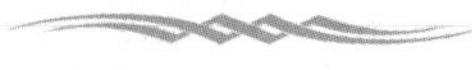

*Appendix C*

# *ETS Plus and Flower Essences*

## ETS PLUS: EMERGENCY TRAUMA SOLUTION

ETS PLUS IS PERELANDRA'S emergency trauma solution that fits everyone's needs for any sudden or long-term traumatic situation. It's a pre-mixed oral solution and easy to take. Just unscrew the dropper cap and take one dose—ten to twelve drops. The range of uses for ETS Plus expands our understanding of trauma. As a result, the many situations throughout these challenging times where our health and well-being are compromised by "traumas" can now be easily addressed.

ETS Plus is especially helpful for stabilizing yourself during a MAP session and immediately after the session for stabilizing your team's work.

ETS Plus can also be taken immediately after taking medications, cutting or burning oneself, feeling overwhelmed in the office, or after a serious accident. For more information about ETS Plus, call our order line or see our web site or catalog.

## WHAT ARE FLOWER ESSENCES AND WHAT DO THEY DO?

The human body has within and surrounding it an electrical network. When we experience health, this electrical network is balanced and fully connected. When something in our life or environment compromises that balance, the corresponding electrical circuits respond by either short-circuiting or overloading. That imbalance in the electrical system immediately impacts the central nervous system and sets up a domino effect within the body that can lead to illness. We can get a cold or a headache, or our allergy pops up again or another migraine belts us. Or we get back pain, our neck goes out, or our arthritis acts up again. Or we become seriously ill.

Flower essences work directly with the electrical system. By taking the correct essences, we balance, stabilize and repair the damaged electrical circuits and stop the domino effect that leads to illness.

If we don't take flower essences and wind up getting sick, the essences will then balance, stabilize and repair the body's electrical circuits while the body gets on with the business of fighting off the problem. By assisting this process, essences will drastically reduce our recovery time.

## THE PERELANDRA ESSENCES

The Perelandra flower essences have been a natural development in the work that has gone on between nature and myself. Carefully prepared from flowers, vegetables and herbs grown in the Perelandra garden, the essences are water-based tinctures that have been infused with specific balancing patterns derived from the petals of the plants. The tinctures go through a final stabilization inside the Genesa® crystal sitting in the center of the garden. They are bottled in *concentrate* form in pharmaceutical dropper bottles that make it easy for you to place one drop of a needed essence on your tongue or several drops of the essence in a glass of water to be sipped throughout the day.

We feel that through these essences we at Perelandra are able to share the extraordinary vitality and power that has resulted from my thirty years working with nature in the Perelandra garden. In using the essences, we establish another partnership with nature—this one focused on our health, balance and well-being.

To learn more about flower essences and how to test them, I recommend the video *The Human Electrical System and Flower Essences.* For more information about this and the Perelandra Essences, call our order line, see our web site or our catalog.

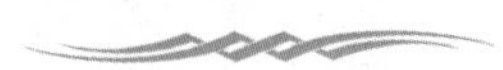

*Appendix D*

# *About Perelandra and My Research with Nature*

PERELANDRA IS BOTH MY HOME and a nature research center. It now consists of forty-five acres of open fields and woods in the foothills of the Blue Ridge Mountains in Virginia. The nature research and development has been going on since 1976, when I dedicated myself to learning about nature in new ways from nature itself. I began working with nature intelligence in a coordinated, co-creative and educational effort that has resulted in a new science called "co-creative science." Traditional science—commonly known as "contemporary science"—is man's study of reality and how it works. Co-creative science is the study of reality and how it works *by man and nature (nature intelligence) working together in a partnership as peers.*

The research at Perelandra focuses on three main areas: environment, health and soil-less gardens (i.e., business, home, the creative arts, special projects—all "gardens" that do not grow in soil.)

Perelandra's main laboratory is its one-hundred-foot-diameter garden. It is here that I work with nature to get the information I need to create an inclusive environment based on nature's principles of balance. We do not use organic or chemical pesticides, herbicides, insecticides or chemical fertilizers. Perelandra's garden laboratory operates according to nature's principles of balance, and it is this information that I get from my nature partner. We have developed guidelines and procedures anyone may use to establish a balanced environment for such diverse areas as a farm, a forest, a ranch, an apartment, a suburban home and yard, a pond or lake, a college dorm, and a business. MAP is just one example of my work with nature in the area of human health.

As I publish this third edition of *MAP* in 2006, I celebrate two big anniversaries. My work with nature began thirty years ago this fall. And Perelandra, as a business and service, began twenty-five years ago. I can honestly say that the past thirty years of working with nature have been an adventure beyond anything I could ever imagine. And I can't imagine where the next thirty years will lead.

To help you understand the work at Perelandra and why nature plays an important and direct role in our health and wellbeing in general, and in MAP and the Calibration Process specifically, I include in Appendix E definitions that were given to me by nature in a coning session. I feel that once you read them you'll sense nature's important role in our life and in human health more clearly.

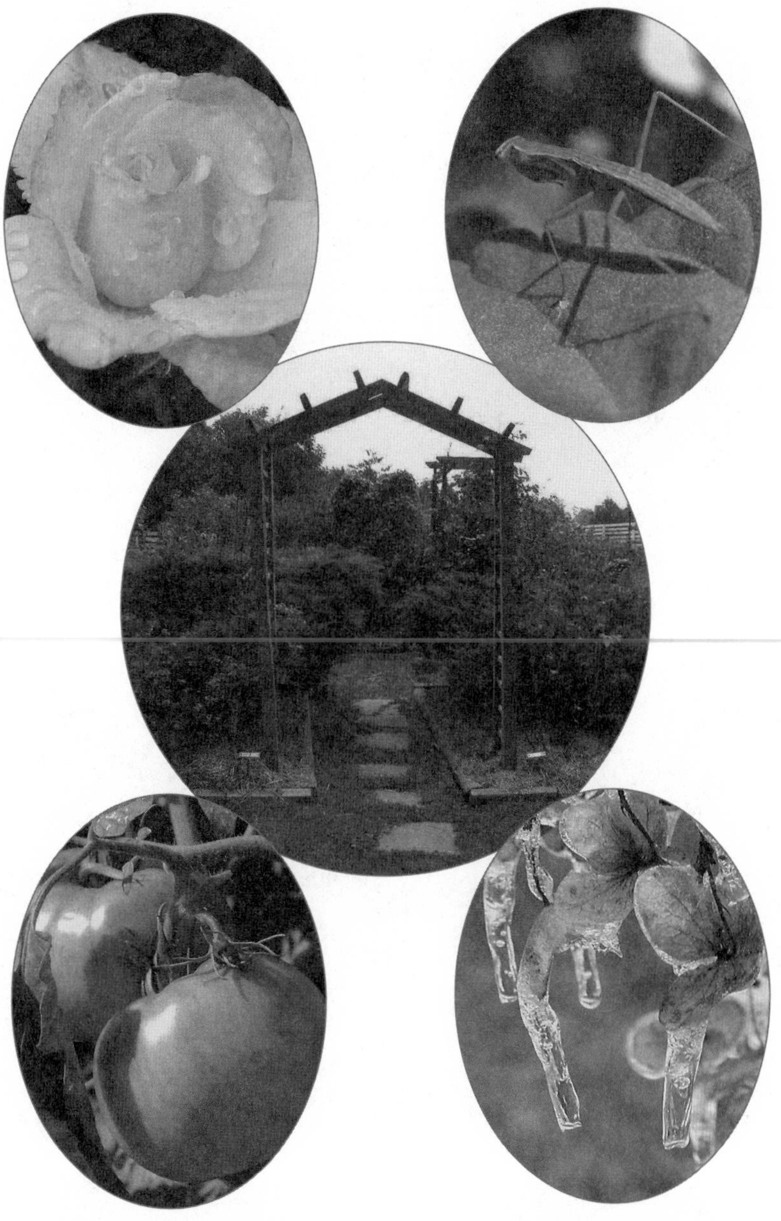

*Scenes from the Perelandra garden.*

*Appendix E*

# *Co-Creative Definitions by Nature and Friends*

*LET US GIVE YOU THE BASIC UNDERSTANDING of these terms. We feel that these definitions, kept short and simple, will be more helpful than lengthy, detailed ones. Consider these definitions to be starting points.*

● FORM. *We consider reality to be in the form state when there is order, organization and life vitality combined with a state of consciousness. For the purpose of understanding form in a constructive and workable manner, let us say that we consider consciousness to be soul-initiated and, therefore, quite capable of function beyond what we would term "form." There are dimensions of reality in which the interaction of life reality is maintained beyond form only. There is no surrounding organization, order, or life vitality as we know it. There is only reality beyond form.*

*We do not consider form to be only that which is perceptible to the five senses. In fact, we see form from this perspective to be most limited, both in its life reality and in its ability to function. We see form from the perspective of the five senses to be useful only for the most basic and fundamental level of identification. From this perspective, there is very little relationship to the full understanding and knowledge of how a unit or form system functions.*

*All energy contains order, organization and life vitality; therefore, all energy is form. If one were to use the term "form" to identify that which can be perceived by the five senses and the word "energy" to refer to that aspect of an animal, human, plant, or object's reality that cannot be readily perceived by the five senses, then one would be accurate in the use of these two words. However, if one were to use the word "form" to refer to that which can be perceived by the five senses and assume form to be a complete unit of reality unto itself, and use the word "energy" to refer to a level beyond form, one would then be using these two words inaccurately.*

*On the planet Earth, the personality, character, emotional make-up, intellectual capacity, strong points and gifts of a human are all form. They are that which gives order, organization and life vitality to consciousness.*

*Order and organization are the physical structures that create a framework for form. In short, they define the walls. But we have included the dynamic of life vitality when we refer to form because one of the elements of form is action, and it is the life vitality that initiates and creates action.*

● NATURE. *In the larger universe and beyond, on its many levels and dimensions, there are a number of groups of consciousnesses that, although equal in importance, are quite different in expression and function. Do not misunderstand us by thinking that we are saying that all reality is human soul-oriented but that there are some aspects of this reality that function and express differently. We are not saying this. We are saying that there are different groups of consciousnesses that are equal in importance but express and function very differently. Together, they make up the full expression of the larger, total life picture. No one piece, no one expression, can be missing or the larger life picture on all its levels and dimensions will cease to exist. One such consciousness has been universally termed "nature." Because of what we are saying about the larger picture not existing without all of its parts, you may assume that nature as both a reality and a consciousness exists on all dimensions and all levels. It cannot be excluded.*

*Each group of consciousnesses has what can be termed an area of expertise. As we said, all groups are equal in importance but express and function differently from one another. These different expressions and functions are vital to the overall balance of reality. A truly symbiotic relationship exists among the groups and is based on balance—universal balance. You are absolutely correct to characterize the human soul-oriented dynamic as evolution in scope and function. And you are correct in identifying the nature dynamic as being involution in scope and function. Nature is a massive, intelligent consciousness group that expresses and functions within the many areas of involution, that is, moving soul-oriented consciousness into any dimension or level of form.*

*Nature is the conscious reality that supplies order, organization and life vitality for this shift. Nature is the consciousness that is, for your working understanding, intimately linked with form. Nature is the consciousness that comprises all form on all levels and dimensions. It is form's order, organization and life vitality. Nature is first and foremost a consciousness of equal importance with all other consciousnesses in the largest scheme of reality. It expresses and functions uniquely in that it comprises all form on all levels and dimensions and is responsible for and creates all of form's order, organization and life vitality.*

● DEVA AND NATURE SPIRIT. *"Devas" and "nature spirit" are names used to identify two different levels and functions within the nature consciousness. They are the two levels within the larger nature consciousness that interface with the human soul while in form. There are other levels, and they are differentiated from one another primarily by specific expression and function.*

*To expand from our definition of form, it is the devic level that fuses with consciousness to create order, organization and life vitality. The devic level as the architect designs the complex order, organization and life vitality that will be needed by the soul consciousness while functioning within the scope or band of form. If the consciousness chooses to shift from one point of form to another point, thereby changing form function, it is the devic level of nature that alters the organization, order and life vitality accordingly. The devic level designs and is the creation of the order, organization and life vitality of form.*

*The nature spirit level infuses the devic order, organization and life vitality and adds to this the dynamic of function and working balance. To order, organization and life vitality it brings movement and the bond that maintains the alignment of the devic form unit to the universal principles of balance while the consciousness is in form.*

*To say that nature is the expert in areas of form and form principles barely scratches the surface of the true nature (pardon the pun) of nature's role in form. It is the expert of form, and it is form itself. A soul-oriented consciousness cannot exist on any level or dimension of form in any way without an equal, intimate, symbiotic relationship with the nature consciousness.*

● CONSCIOUSNESS. *The concept of consciousness has been vastly misunderstood. To put it simply, consciousness is the working state of the soul. In human expression, as one sees it demonstrated on the planet Earth, the personality, character, emotional makeup, intellectual capacity, strong points and gifts of a human are all form. They are that which gives order, organization and life vitality to consciousness.*

*We say "working state of the soul" because there are levels of soul existence that are different than the working state and can best be described as a simple and complete state of being. The closest that souls on Earth come to this notion is the state of unconsciousness. But this is to give you a glimpse of what we mean by "state of being." We urge you not to assume that what you know as unconsciousness is equal to the soul state of being.*

*Humans tend to think of the soul as being something that exists far away from them because they are in form. This is an illusion. The core of any life is the soul. It cannot exist apart from itself. Like the heart in the human body, it is an essential part of the life unit. A human in form is, by definition, a soul fused with nature. Personality and character are a part of the nature/form package that allows the soul to function and to express itself in form. They are not the soul; they are the order and organization of that soul.*

*Consciousness physically fuses into the body system first through the electrical system and then through the central nervous system and the brain. This is another aspect of nature supplying order, organization and life vitality. Consciousness itself cannot be measured or monitored as a reality. But what can be measured and monitored is the order, organization and life vitality of consciousness. Consciousness is the working state of the soul and is not form. It is nature, not consciousness, that supplies form.*

*We wish to add a thought here so that there will be no confusion about the relationship between nature and the soul. The devic level of nature does not, with its own power, superimpose its interpretation of form onto a soul. We have said that nature and soul are intimately and symbiotically related. This implies a give and take.*

*No one consciousness group operates in isolation of the whole or of all other parts of the whole. When a soul chooses to move within the vast band of form, it communicates its intent and purpose to nature. It is from this that nature, on the devic level, derives the specifics that will be needed for the soul to function in form. It is a perfect marriage of purpose with the order, organization and life vitality that is needed for the fulfillment of that purpose. Nature, therefore, does not define purpose and impose it on a soul. It orders, organizes and gives life vitality to purpose for expression of form.*

● SOUL. *We perceive that most likely the question of soul will arise with anyone reading these definitions. This will be most difficult to define since the soul is, at its point of central essence, beyond form. Consequently, it is beyond words. However, it is not beyond any specific life form. As we have said, an individual is not separate or distant from his or her soul. Souls, as individuated life forces, were created in form at the moment you call the "Big Bang." Beyond form, souls are also beyond the notion of creation. So we refer to the moment of the Big Bang regarding the soul, since this gives you a description of soul that will be most meaningful to you.*

*The Big Bang was the nature-designed order, organization and life force used to differentiate soul into sparks of individuated light energy. The power of the Big Bang was created by intent. And that intent originated from the massive collective soul reality beyond form.*

*It is reasonable to look at the Big Bang as the soul's gateway to the immense band of form. To perceive the soul and how it functions exclusively from the perspective of human form on Earth is akin to seeing that planet from the perspective of one grain of sand.*

*The soul's options of function and expression in form are endless. What we see occurring more frequently now on Earth is the shift from the individual soul unknowingly functioning in an array of options, all chosen only because they are compatible to the immediate purpose of the soul, to the individual beginning to function with discrimination and intent in more expanded ways. Using the words in their more limited, parochial definitions, we can say that we see the beginning of a shift from soul function in which an individuated personality remains unaware of many of its options to soul function in which the personality begins to take on conscious awareness of all its options.*

● ENERGY. *For those experiencing life on Earth, energy is form that is perceived by an individual beyond the scope of the basic five senses. All energy contains order, organization and life vitality; therefore, all energy is form. The makeup and design of the specific order, organization and life vitality within that which can be perceived by the basic five senses is identical to and therefore harmonious with its broader reality, which cannot be perceived by the basic five senses. If one is to use the term "form" to identify that which can be perceived by the basic senses and the word "energy" to refer to that aspect of an animal, human, plant, or object's reality that cannot be readily perceived by the basic senses, then one would be accurate in the use of these two words. However, if one is to use the word "form" to refer to that which can be perceived by the basic five senses and assume form to be a complete unit of reality unto itself and use the word "energy" to refer to a level beyond form, one would then be using these two words inaccurately. From our perspective, form and energy create one unit of reality and are differentiated from one another solely by the individual's ability to perceive them with his or her sensory system. In short, the differen-*

*tiation between form and energy within any given object, plant, animal, or human lies with the observer.*

● BASIC SENSORY SYSTEM PERCEPTION. *We define basic sensory system perception as being that which the vast majority of individuals on Earth experience. The acts of seeing, hearing, touching, tasting and smelling fall within what we acknowledge as a basic, fundamental range of sensory development that is predominant on the Earth level. What is referred to as an "expansion experience" is, in fact, an act or experience that is perceived by an individual because of an expansion of the range in which his sensory system operates. Expansion experiences are not perceived outside or beyond an individual's electrical system, central nervous system and sensory system. These three systems are interrelated, and an accurate perception of an expansion experience requires that the three systems operate in concert. Therefore, it is quite possible for something to occur in an individual's life that registers in the person's electrical system and central nervous system but then short-circuits, is altered, or is blocked simply because the person's present sensory system does not have the ability to process, due to its present range of operation, what has registered in the other two systems. People say that "these kinds of strange things never happen to me." This is inaccurate. "Strange" things, experiences and moments beyond the present state of their sensory systems are continuously happening around them and to them. They are simply not at the point where their sensory systems are capable of clear, useful processing. They waste time by directing their will and focus to "make things happen." That is useless since things are happening all the time around them. Instead they should relax and continue through an organic developmental process that is already in effect and that will gradually allow them to accurately perceive what is happening around them. In some cases where events or experiences are vaguely perceived or processed in outrageous, useless ways, their sensory system is expanding but still not operating within the range where events can be usefully processed.*

● REALITY. *From our perspective, reality refers to all levels and dimensions of life experience within form and beyond form. Reality does not depend on an individual's perception of it in order to exist. We call an individual's perception of reality his "perceived reality." Any life system that was created in form (which occurred at the moment of the Big Bang) has inherent in it all dimensions and levels that exist both within form and beyond. How we relate to an individual or object depends on our present ability to enfold and envelop an individual's many levels. The scope within which one exists, the reality of one's existence, is truly beyond form, beyond description. If one understands that the evolutionary force that moves all life systems forward is endless—beyond time—then one must also consider that it is the continuous discovery of these vast levels inherent in all life systems that creates that evolutionary momentum. Since that dynamic is beyond time as expressed on any form level or dimension, it is endless.*

● PERCEIVED REALITY. *This is the combination of elements that make up an individual's full system of reality and are perceived, embraced and enfolded by him or by another individual at any given time. From this, an individual "knows" himself or another individual only from the perspective of the specific combination of elements he or she is able to perceive, embrace and enfold. Any one element can be considered a window to the larger whole. When in form, these elements take on the dynamics of order, organization and life vitality and are demonstrated through these specific form frameworks. The extent to which perceived reality corresponds to the larger, all-encompassing reality depends on the ability of an individual to accurately demonstrate these elements within form frameworks and the ability of that or another individual to accurately perceive what is being demonstrated.*

● BALANCE. *Balance is relative and measured, shall we say, by an individual's ability to faithfully demonstrate the various elements that make up his larger reality through the specific frameworks of form in which one has chosen to develop. When what one is demonstrating is faithful in intent and clarity with these elements and the larger reality, one experiences balance. And those interacting with this individual will experience his balance. One experiences imbalance when there is distortion between what one demonstrates through the form framework and the intent and clarity of the elements that make up the larger reality as well as the larger reality itself.*

*If you seriously consider what we are saying here, you will see that balance as a phenomenon is not an elusive state that only an exalted few can achieve. Balance is, in fact, inherent in all reality, in all life systems. Balance is defined by the many elements within any individual's reality. And it is the dominant state of being within any reality and any form system. It is also the state of being that links individual life systems to one another and to the larger whole. When one says that he is a child of the universe, what one is acknowledging is the relationship and link of his higher state of balance to the universe's state of balance. Whether he feels linked to or distant from this relationship depends on the closeness or distance he creates within himself with respect to his larger personal state of balance—that dynamic that is part of his overall reality.*

● LIFE VITALITY. *We have used this term frequently in these definitions and feel it would be useful to clarify what we mean. To understand life vitality, it is best to see it in relationship to order and organization. Order and organization are the physical structures that create the framework for form. In short, they define the walls. But we have included the dynamic of life vitality when we refer to form because one element of form is action, and it is life vitality that initiates and creates action. Nothing in form is stagnant. It is life vitality that gives to form its action. If the framework that is created from order and organization is incomplete, ineffective, deteriorating or being dismantled in an untimely manner, the dynamic of life vitality decreases within the overall form reality. This causes life movement to decrease accordingly, and is a movement toward a state of stagnation. It is the dynamic of vitality that gives life—movement—to any individual or object. Organization and order alone cannot do that. However, vitality without organization and order has no sense of purpose to its motion. It cannot function without organization and order. The three must be present and in balance with one another for there to be quality form expression. Nature, on the devic level, creates organization, order and life vitality in perfect balance. Nature, on the nature spirit level, maintains that balanced relationship as individual life units move through their evolutionary paces.*

*We would like to illustrate what we are saying by focusing your attention on the soil-balancing process that improves and enhances the level of soil vitality. This process does not work directly with the soil's vitality level. Instead, it works with those elements of the soil that constitute its order and organization. This balancing process shores up the physical structure of its order and organization. As a direct result, the soil begins to shift its form back to the original balance among organization, order and life vitality. As a consequence of this shift, the soil vitality level (the soil's life vitality) increases to its new state of balance. Those changes involve a comparable shift in the interaction and movement among all the different elements that make up soil. This is why when someone observes change in a field that has had its soil balanced through the soil-balancing process, he sees greater efficiency between how the soil and plants interact. The action and movement in the soil have raised the soil's order and organizational structures back to the state (or nearer to the state) of the original devic balance of order, organization and life vitality.*

● GROUNDING. *Quite simply, the word "grounded" is used to acknowledge full body/soul fusion or full matter/soul fusion. The word "grounding" refers to what must be accomplished or activated in order to both ensure and stabilize body or matter/soul fusion. To be grounded refers to the state of being a fused body (matter)/soul unit. To achieve this unit fusion and to function fully as a fused unit is the primary goal one accepts when choosing to experience life within form. Functioning as a grounded body (matter)/soul unit is a goal on all levels and dimensions of form, whether the form can or cannot be perceived by the five senses.*

*Nature plays two key roles in grounding. First, it is through and with nature that the grounding occurs. Nature, which organizes, orders and adds life vitality to create form, is what creates and maintains grounding. Second, the levels of nature know what is required to fuse the soul dynamic within form. Nature provides the best examples of body (matter)/soul fusion. Humans have recognized the form or matter existence of nature on the planet, but have only recently begun to understand that within all form there are fully functioning soul dynamics. On the other hand, humans acknowledge or concentrate on their personal soul dynamics but have little understanding as to how they, in order to be functional within form, must allow the soul to fuse with and operate through their form body. Humans do not see the examples or learn the lessons of the master teachers of body (matter)/soul fusion that surround them in all the kingdoms of nature. Humans also deny the fusion within themselves. The relative extent of this denial interferes proportionately with the quality and stabilization of the fusion.*

● INTENT. *Intent refers to the conscious dynamic within all life that links life vitality with soul purpose and direction. When an individual uses free will to manipulate what he or she willfully desires instead of what is within the scope of higher soul purpose, then intent is combined with the manipulative power of free will and this combination is linked with life vitality. If you will recall, it is life vitality that adds action to order and organization. It both initiates and creates action. To maintain harmonious movement with soul purpose and direction, life vitality must be linked with the soul dynamic. This linkage occurs on two levels. One is unconscious, allowing for a natural patterning and rhythm of action through form that is consistent with soul purpose. As the body/soul fusion moves through its own evolutionary process as a functioning unit, it takes on a greater level of consciousness and an expanded level of awareness and knowing. As a result, the unconscious link between soul dynamic and life vitality takes on a new level of operation, thus shifting it into a state of consciousness. The shift is a gradual, step-by-step evolutionary process in itself. Intent is conscious awareness of soul purpose, what is required within the scope of form to achieve soul purpose, and how the two function as a unit. Consequently, when one wishes to express soul purpose, one need only consciously fuse this purpose with appropriate form and action. This act is what is referred to when one speaks of intent.*

*Intent as a dynamic is an evolutionary process in itself and, as we have said, does not suddenly envelop one's entire life fully and completely. Intent is only gradually incorporated into one's everyday life. Therefore, one does not suddenly and immediately function within the full scope of the intent dynamic in those areas of life where intent is present. Intent as a dynamic is as broad a learning arena as life itself. And in the beginning, intent can often be confused with or intermingled with free will. However, as it is developed, it becomes the cutting edge of the body/soul unit and how it operates. Intent is the key to unlimited life within the scope of form.*

● INTUITION. *Intuition, as it is popularly defined, relates to a sixth sense of operation. This is false. This is not a sixth sense. When individuals experience a phenomenon that they consider to be beyond their five senses, they tend to attribute this experience to another category, the sixth sense, and call it intuition. The fact is that these expanded experiences are processed through their five senses in an expanded manner.*

*Intuition, in fact, is related to and linked with intent. It is the bridge between an individual's conscious body/soul fusion—that state which he knows and understands about the body/soul fusion and how it functions—and the individual's unconscious body/soul fusion. The intuition bridges the unconscious and the conscious. This enables what is known on the level of the unconscious body/soul fusion to be incorporated with and become a part of the conscious body/soul fusion. Intuition is the communication bridge between the two that makes it possible for the conscious body/soul unit to benefit from those aspects of the unconscious body/soul unit. This benefit results when the conscious unit opens to and moves through the lessons surrounding intent. Where intent is functioning fully, these two levels, the unconscious and the conscious, are no longer separate but have become one—the expanded conscious level. Consequently, there is then no need for the bridge known as intuition.*

*However, lest you think otherwise, intent is not considered greater than intuition; rather, they are two excellent tools utilized equally by the highest developed souls functioning within form. We say this to caution those who read this not to think intent is "greater" than intuition and to be aimed for at the exclusion of intuition. Evolution as seen from the highest perspective is endless. Therefore, discovery of all there is to know about both intuition and intent is endless. For all practical purposes, an individual can safely consider that there will never be a time in which the development of intent will be such that the need for and development of intuition will be unnecessary. As we have said, the highest souls who function to the fullest within the scope of form do so with an equal development and expansion of both intent and intuition.*

## BOOKS BY MACHAELLE WRIGHT

*Behaving as if the God in All Life Mattered*
Third Edition, 1997

*Co-Creative Science:*
*A Revolution in Science Providing Real Solutions for Todays Health and Environment*
First Edition, 1997

*Dancing in the Shadows of the Moon*
First Edition, 1995

*The Mount Shasta Mission*
First Edition, 2005

*The Perelandra Essences:*
*A Revolution in Our Understanding and Approach to Illness and Health*
First Edition, 2011

*MAP:*
*The Co-Creative White Brotherhood Medical Assistance Program*
Third Edition, 2006

*Perelandra Microbial Balancing Program Manual*
Second Edition, 2004

*The Perelandra Garden Workbook*
First Edition, 2012

*Perelandra Soil-less Garden Companion*
First Edition, 2007

PERELANDRA, LTD.
P.O. Box 3603
Warrenton, VA 20188

U.S. & Canada Order Line: 1-800-960-8806
Overseas & Mexico Order Line: 1-540-937-2153
Question Hot Line: 1-540-937-3679
Fax: 1-540-937-3360
Web Site: www.perelandra-ltd.com
E-mail: email@perelandra-ltd.com

## PERELANDRA PHONE ORDER LINE

The nice folks in our customer service department can answer questions about the products, help you figure what to order and tell you the most economical way to order it.

## PERELANDRA WEB SITE

You can also visit our beautiful, extensive and user-friendly web site. Along with browsing our complete and up-to-date catalog or placing an order, you can visit our Education section for answers to frequently asked questions, excerpts from each of our books or one of the many informative articles. Overall, our goal is for the web site to be as much a resource and education center as it is an online catalog. It also includes money-saving specials, networking lists, a weekly photo gallery of the Perelandra garden, and special health and product updates.

## PERELANDRA CATALOG

Information about Perelandra and descriptions of Perelandra products are included in our free catalog. Our catalog is available upon request.

## PERELANDRA QUESTION HOT LINE

Get your questions answered about any of the processes and Perelandra tools. Call our order line or see our web site or catalog for the Question Hot Line hours.

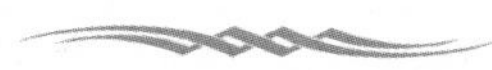